The Respiratory System at a Glance

The Respiratory System at a Glance

Jeremy P.T. Ward

PhD
Head of Department of Physiology
and Professor of Respiratory Cell Physiology
Division of Asthma, Allergy and Lung Biology
King's College London
London, UK

Jane Ward

MBChB, PhD
Senior Lecturer
Department of Physiology
King's College London
London, UK

Richard M. Leach

MD, FRCP
Consultant Physician and Honorary Senior Lecturer
Guy's and St Thomas' Hospital Trust and
King's College London School of Medicine
St Thomas' Hospital
London, UK

With contributions from

Charles M. Wiener

MD
Professor of Medicine and Physiology
Department of Medicine
Johns Hopkins School of Medicine
Baltimore MD, USA

Third edition

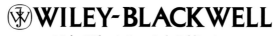

A John Wiley & Sons, Ltd., Publication

This edition first published 2010, © 2010 by J.P.T. Ward, J. Ward, R.M. Leach
Previous editions: 2002, 2006

Blackwell Publishing was acquired by John Wiley & Sons in February 2007. Blackwell's publishing program has been merged with Wiley's global Scientific, Technical and Medical business to form Wiley-Blackwell.

Registered office: John Wiley & Sons Ltd, The Atrium, Southern Gate, Chichester, West Sussex, PO19 8SQ, UK

Editorial offices: 9600 Garsington Road, Oxford, OX4 2DQ, UK
    The Atrium, Southern Gate, Chichester, West Sussex, PO19 8SQ, UK
    111 River Street, Hoboken, NJ 07030-5774, USA

For details of our global editorial offices, for customer services and for information about how to apply for permission to reuse the copyright material in this book please see our website at www.wiley.com/wiley-blackwell

Library of Congress Cataloging-in-Publication Data

Ward, Jeremy P. T.
   The respiratory system at a glance / Jeremy P.T. Ward, Jane Ward, and Richard M. Leach ; with contributions by Charles M. Weiner. – 3rd ed.
       p. ; cm. – (At a glance)
   Includes index.
   Rev. ed. of: Respiratory system at a glance / Jeremy P.T. Ward . . . [et al.]. 2006.
   ISBN 978-1-4051-9919-3
   1. Respiratory organs–Diseases.   I. Ward, Jane, MBChB.   II. Leach, Richard M., MD.   III. Title.
IV. Series: At a glance series (Oxford, England).
   [DNLM: 1. Respiratory Physiological Phenomena.   2. Respiratory System–physiopathology.
3. Respiratory Tract Diseases. WF 102 W259r 2010]
   RC731.R493 2010
   616.2–dc22

                                                                    2010015122

ISBN: 9781405199193

A catalogue record for this book is available from the British Library.

Set in 9/11.5pt Times by Aptara® Inc., New Delhi, India
Printed in Singapore by Markono Print Media Pte Ltd

2   2011

Contents

Preface to third edition

The medical curriculum has become increasingly vertically integrated, with a much greater use of clinical examples and cases to help in the understanding of the relevance of the underlying basic science, and conversely use of basic science concepts to help in the understanding of the pathophysiology and treatment of disease. *The Respiratory System at a Glance* has been written to take account of this trend, and to integrate core aspects of basic science, pathophysiology and treatment into a single, easy to use revision aid. As such, it should be useful to medical students throughout their training, and also to other healthcare professions, including nursing.

As with other volumes in the *At a Glance* series, it is based around a two-page spread for each main topic, with figures and text complementing each other to give an overview of a topic at a glance. Case studies based on some of the most commonly encountered conditions are also provided, and can be used for both basic science and clinical study. Although primarily designed for revision, the book covers all the core elements of the respiratory system and its major diseases, and as such could be used as a main text in the first couple of years of the course. It is advised, however, that additional reference to more detailed textbooks will aid deeper and wider understanding of the subject. This is particularly the case for the pathophysiological chapters, as a book of this length cannot hope to provide a complete guide to clinical practice.

The most notable change to this third edition is that the figures are now in colour, which should aid understanding. There are also new or expanded sections on topics such as public health and smoking, sarcoidosis and sleep-disordered breathing, additional case studies and self-assessment MCQs. Most of the other chapters and figures have been revised and updated. Hopefully, we have also corrected remaining errors found in the last edition. We have been greatly assisted in this by our many colleagues and students who have kindly advised us and commented on the contents, but any remaining errors and omissions are entirely our responsibility. We also thank all the staff at Wiley-Blackwell, without whom we would not have been able to produce this edition on time.

Jeremy P.T. Ward
Jane Ward
Richard M. Leach

Units and symbols

Units

The medical profession and scientific community generally use SI (Système International) units.

Pressure conversion: SI unit of pressure: 1 pascal (Pa) $= 1\,N \cdot m^{-2}$. As this is small, in medicine the kPa ($=10^3$ Pa) is more commonly used. Note that millimetres of mercury (mmHg) are still the most common unit for expressing arterial and venous blood pressures, and low pressures – e.g. central venous pressure and intrapleural pressure – are sometimes expressed as centimetres of H_2O (cmH_2O). Blood gas partial pressures are reported by some laboratories in kPa and by some in mmHg, so you need to be familiar with both systems.

1 kPa = 7.5 mmHg = 10.2 cmH_2O

1 mmHg = 1 torr = 0.133 kPa = 1.36 cmH_2O

1 cmH_2O = 0.098 kPa = 0.74 mmHg

1 standard atmosphere ($\approx$1 bar) = 101.3 kPa = 760 mmHg = 1033 cmH_2O

Contents are still commonly expressed per 100 mL (dL^{-1}), and these need to be multiplied by 10 to give the more standard SI unit per litre. Contents are also increasingly being expressed as $mmol \cdot L^{-1}$.

For haemoglobin: $1\,g \cdot dL^{-1} = 10\,g \cdot L^{-1} = 0.062\,mmol \cdot L^{-1}$

For ideal gases (including oxygen and nitrogen): 1 mmol = 22.4 mL standard temperature and pressure dry (STPD; see Chapter 4)

For non-ideal gases, such as nitrous oxide and carbon dioxide: 1 mmol = 22.25 mL STPD

Standard symbols

Primary symbols

F = Fractional concentration of gas

C = Content of a gas in blood

V = Volume of a gas

P = Pressure of partial pressure

S = Saturation of haemoglobin with oxygen

Q = Volume of blood

A dot over a letter means a time derivative, e.g. $\dot{V}$ = ventilation (L/min); $\dot{Q}$ = blood flow (L/min)

Secondary symbols

Gas:
I = Inspired gas
E = Expired gas
A = Alveolar gas
D = Dead-space gas
T = Tidal
B = Barometric
ET = End-tidal

Blood:
a = Arterial
v = Venous
c = Capillary
A dash means mixed or mean
e.g. $\bar{v}$ = Mixed venous
A' after a symbol means end
e.g. c' = End-capillary

Tertiary symbols

O_2 = Oxygen

CO_2 = Carbon dioxide

CO = Carbon monoxide

Examples

$\dot{V}O_2$ = Oxygen consumption

P_ACO_2 = Alveolar partial pressure of carbon dioxide

Typical values

Typical inspired, alveolar and blood gas values in healthy young adults are shown in the table below. Ranges are given for arterial blood gas values. Mean arterial PO_2 falls with age, and by 60 years is about 11 kPa/82 mmHg. Typical values for lung volumes and other lung function tests are given in the appropriate chapters. Ranges for many values are affected by age, sex and height, as well as by the method of measurement, and hence it is necessary to refer to appropriate nomograms.

Inspired PO_2 (dry, sea level)	21 kPa	159 mmHg
Alveolar PO_2	13.3 kPa	100 mmHg
Arterial PO_2	12.5 (11.2–13.9) kPa	94 (84–104) mmHg
A–a PO_2 gradient	<2 kPa	<15 mmHg (greater in elderly)
Arterial oxygen saturation	>97%	
Arterial oxygen content	$200\,mL \cdot L^{-1}$	$20\,mL \cdot dL^{-1}$
Inspired PCO_2	0.03 kPa	0.2 mmHg
Alveolar PCO_2	5.3 (4.7–6.1) kPa	40 (35–45) mmHg
Arterial PCO_2	5.3 (4.7–6.1) kPa	40 (35–45) mmHg
Arterial CO_2 content	$480\,mL \cdot L^{-1}$	$48\,mL \cdot dL^{-1}$
Arterial $[H^+]$/pH	36–$44\,nmol \cdot L^{-1}$	7.44–7.36
Resting mixed venous PO_2	5.3 kPa	40 mmHg
Resting mixed venous O_2 content	$150\,mL \cdot L^{-1}$	$15\,mL \cdot dL^{-1}$
Resting mixed venous O_2 saturation	75%	
Resting mixed venous PCO_2	6.1 kPa	46 mmHg
Resting mixed venous CO_2 content	$520\,mL \cdot L^{-1}$	$52\,mL \cdot dL^{-1}$
Arterial $[HCO_3^-]$	24 (21–27) mM	

List of abbreviations

A–a gradient	$(A–a\ Po_2)$ gradient, the difference between ideal alveolar and arterial Po_2	**DVT**	deep venous thrombosis
AAT	α_1-antitrypsin	**EBV**	Epstein–Barr virus
AHI	apnoea plus hypopnoea index	**ECG**	electrocardiogram
AIDS	acquired immune deficiency syndrome	**ECMO**	extracorporeal membrane oxygenation
AIP	acute interstitial pneumonia/pneumonitis (Hamman–Rich syndrome)	**ECP**	eosinophil cationic protein
ALI	acute lung injury	**EEG**	electroencephalogram
ANA	anti-nuclear antibody	**EGF**	epidermal growth factor
ANCA	anti-neutrophil cytoplasmic antibody	**ELISA**	enzyme-linked immunoassay
AP	anterior–posterior	**EMG**	electromyogram
ARDS	acute (formerly adult) respiratory distress syndrome	**EOG**	electrooculogram
ATPS	ambient temperature and pressure saturated	**ERV**	expiratory reserve volume
ATS	American Thoracic Society (guidelines)	**ESR**	erythrocyte sedimentation rate
BAL	bronchoalveolar lavage	**FDG**	fluorodeoxyglucose
BALT	bronchus-associated lymphoid tissue	**FDG PET**	fluorodeoxyglucose positron emission tomography
BCG	bacille Calmette–Guérin	**FEF$_{25-75}$**	mean forced expiratory flow over middle 50% of forced vital capacity
BiPAP	bilevel positive airway pressure, biphasic positive airway pressure	**FER**	forced expiratory ratio
BP	blood pressure	**FEV$_1$**	forced expiratory volume in 1 second
BTPS	body temperature and pressure saturated	**FEV$_1$/FVC**	FEV_1 expressed as a fraction, or more usually a percentage of FVC (= FER)
BTS	British Thoracic Society (guidelines)	**FGF**	fibroblast growth factor
CA	carbonic anhydrase	**FRC**	functional residual capacity
cAMP	cyclic adenosine monophosphate	**FVC**	forced vital capacity
CAP	community-acquired pneumonia	**GBM**	glomerular basement membrane
CCF	congestive cardiac failure	**GM-CSF**	granulocyte macrophage colony-stimulating factor
CF	cystic fibrosis	**GU**	genitourinary
CFA	cryptogenic fibrosing alveolitis	**HAART**	highly active antiretroviral therapy
CFTR	cystic fibrosis transmembrane conductance regulator	**HAP**	hospital acquired pneumonia
C$_L$	lung compliance = $\Delta V/\Delta P$, where P = alveolar – intrapleural pressure	**HCAP**	healthcare-associated pneumonia
		HIV	human immunodeficiency virus
CMV	controlled mechanical ventilation	**HR**	heart rate
CMV	cytomegalovirus	**HRCT**	high-resolution computed tomography
CNS	central nervous system	**ICU**	intensive care unit
COAD	chronic obstructive airway disease (synonymous with COPD, COLD)	**IFN-γ**	interferon-γ
		Ig	immunoglobulin, e.g. IgA, IgE, IgG and IgM
COLD	chronic obstructive lung disease (synonymous with COAD, COPD)	**IL**	interleukin, e.g. IL-10
		ILD	interstitial lung disease
COPD	chronic obstructive pulmonary disease (synonymous with COAD, COLD)	**INPV**	intermittent negative pressure ventilation
		IPF	idiopathic pulmonary fibrosis (synonymous with CFA)
COX	cyclooxygenase		
CPAP	continuous positive airway pressure	**IPPV**	intermittent positive pressure breathing
CREST	calcinosis, Raynaud's phenomenon, esophageal involvement, sclerodactyly and telangiectasia	**IRV**	inspiratory reserve volume
		IVC	inferior vena cava
		JVP	jugular venous pressure
CSA	central sleep apnoea	**K$_{CO}$**	D_LCO divided by alveolar volume or Krough coefficient
CSF	cerebrospinal fluid		
CT	computed tomography	**KS**	Kaposi's sarcoma
CTPA	computed tomography pulmonary angiogram	**LA**	left atrium, left atrial
CWP	coal worker's pneumoconiosis	**LDH**	lactate dehydrogenase
CXR	chest X-ray	**LG**	lymphomatoid granulomatosis
DIP	desquamative interstitial pneumonia	**LIP**	lymphocytic interstitial pneumonia
D$_L$CO	diffusing capacity of the lungs for carbon monoxide	**LMWH**	low-molecular-weight heparin
D$_L$g	diffusing capacity of the lungs for gas	**LT**	leukotriene, e.g. LTC$_4$
D$_L$O$_2$	diffusing capacity of the lungs for oxygen	**LV**	left ventricle, left ventricular
DRG	dorsal respiratory group	**MBP**	major basic protein

MDR	multidrug resistant	**PPHN**	persistent pulmonary hypertension of the newborn
MI	myocardial infarction	**PSP**	primary spontaneous pneumothorax
MIE	meconium ileus equivalent	**R**	respiratory gas exchange ratio
MMV	mandatory minute ventilation	**RAD**	right axis deviation (electrocardiography)
MOF	multiorgan failure	**RANTES**	regulated on activation normal T cell expressed and secreted
MRSA	methicillin-resistant *Staphylococcus aureus*	**RAW**	airway resistance (mouth–alveolar pressure/airflow)
MVV	maximal voluntary ventilation	**RBBB**	right bundle-branch block
NANC	non-adrenergic, non-cholinergic (nerves)	**RBC**	red blood cell
NHL	non-Hodgkin's lymphoma	**REM**	rapid eye movement
NIPPV	non-invasive positive pressure ventilation	**RV**	residual volume
NRDS	neonatal respiratory distress syndrome	**RV**	right ventricle
NREM	non-rapid eye movement	**RVD**	restrictive ventilatory defect
NSAID	non-steroidal anti-inflammatory drug	$S_{a}o_2$	oxygen saturation of arterial blood (%)
NSC	non-small cell	**SC**	small cell
NSIP	non-specific interstitial pneumonia	**SCUBA**	self-contained underwater breathing apparatus
OSA	obstructive sleep apnoea	**SIADH**	syndrome of inappropriate secretion of antidiuretic hormone
P_{50}	partial pressure at which haemoglobin is 50% saturated with O_2	**SIMV**	synchronized intermittent mandatory ventilation
P_A	alveolar pressure	**SLE**	systemic lupus erythematosus
PA	posterior–anterior	So_2	oxygen saturation (oxygen content/oxygen capacity)
PA	pulmonary arterial	**SP**	surfactant protein, e.g. SP-A
P_Aco	partial pressure of carbon monoxide in the alveoli	**STPD**	standard temperature and pressure dry
$P_{a}co_2$	arterial partial pressure of carbon dioxide	**SVC**	superior vena cava
$P_{A}co_2$	alveolar partial pressure of CO_2	**TB**	tuberculosis
PAF	platelet-activating factor	**TGF**β	transforming growth factor β
PAH	pulmonary arterial hypertension	**TLC**	total lung capacity
$P_{a}o_2$	partial pressure of oxygen in the arterial blood	T_Lco	carbon monoxide transfer factor (alternative name for D_Lco)
PCP	*Pneumocystis carinii* pneumonia	**UFH**	unfractionated heparin
$PD_{20}FEV_1$	provocative dose (e.g. of histamine or methacholine) that induces a 20% fall in FEV_1	**UIP**	usual interstitial pneumonia
PDGF	platelet-derived growth factor	**VAP**	ventilator-associated pneumonia
PE	pulmonary embolus, pulmonary embolism	V_A/Q	ventilation–perfusion ratio (alveolar ventilation/blood flow in a lung region)
PEEP	positive end-expiratory pressure	**VC**	vital capacity
PEFR	peak expiratory flow rate	**VEGF**	vascular endothelial growth factor
PET	positron emission tomography	**VIP**	vasoactive intestinal peptide
Pg	prostaglandin, e.g. PgD_2	$\dot{V}o_2max$	maximum oxygen consumption
PH	pulmonary hypertension	**VRG**	ventral respiratory groups
pHa	arterial pH	V_T	tidal volume
pK_A	log of dissociation constant K_A	**WBC**	white blood cell
PMF	progressive massive fibrosis	**WCC**	white cell count
PMI	point of maximal impulse (also known as Apex beat)	**WG**	Wegener's granulomatosis
PPD	purified protein derivative		

Structure of the respiratory system: lungs, airways and dead space

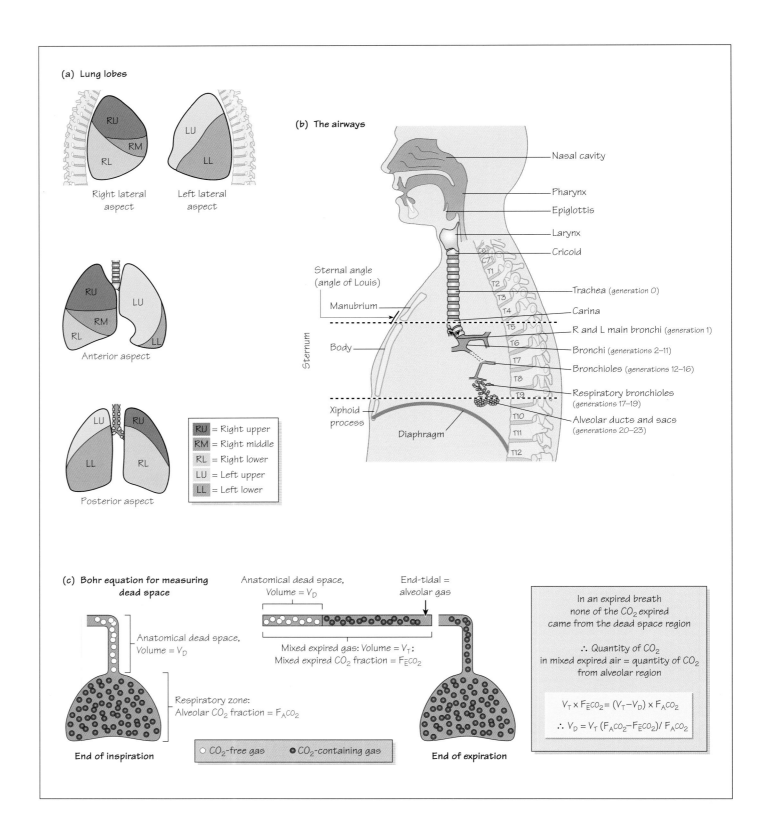

(a) Lung lobes

Right lateral aspect   Left lateral aspect

Anterior aspect

Posterior aspect

RU = Right upper
RM = Right middle
RL = Right lower
LU = Left upper
LL = Left lower

(b) The airways

Nasal cavity
Pharynx
Epiglottis
Larynx
Cricoid

Sternal angle (angle of Louis)
Manubrium
Sternum
Body
Xiphoid process
Diaphragm

Trachea (generation 0)
Carina
R and L main bronchi (generation 1)
Bronchi (generations 2–11)
Bronchioles (generations 12–16)
Respiratory bronchioles (generations 17–19)
Alveolar ducts and sacs (generations 20–23)

(c) Bohr equation for measuring dead space

Anatomical dead space, Volume = V_D

End-tidal = alveolar gas

Anatomical dead space, Volume = V_D

Mixed expired gas: Volume = V_T; Mixed expired CO_2 fraction = $F_E CO_2$

Respiratory zone: Alveolar CO_2 fraction = $F_A CO_2$

○ CO_2-free gas   ● CO_2-containing gas

End of inspiration   End of expiration

In an expired breath none of the CO_2 expired came from the dead space region

∴ Quantity of CO_2 in mixed expired air = quantity of CO_2 from alveolar region

$$V_T \times F_E CO_2 = (V_T - V_D) \times F_A CO_2$$

$$\therefore V_D = V_T (F_A CO_2 - F_E CO_2)/ F_A CO_2$$

Lungs

The respiratory system consists of a pair of **lungs** within the **thoracic cage** (Chapter 2). Its main function is gas exchange, but other roles include speech, filtration of microthrombi arriving from systemic veins and metabolic activities such as conversion of angiotensin I to angiotensin II and removal or deactivation of serotonin, bradykinin, norepinephrine, acetylcholine and drugs such as propranolol and chlorpromazine. The **right lung** is divided by **transverse** and **oblique fissures** into three lobes: upper, middle and lower. The **left lung** has an **oblique fissure** and two lobes (Fig. 1a). Vessels, nerves and lymphatics enter the lungs on their medial surfaces at the lung root or **hilum**. Each lobe is divided into a number of wedge-shaped **bronchopulmonary segments** with their apices at the hilum and bases at the lung surface. Each bronchopulmonary segment is supplied by its own segmental bronchus, artery and vein and can be removed surgically with little bleeding or air leakage from the remaining lung.

The **pulmonary nerve plexus** lies behind each hilum, receiving fibres from both **vagi** and the second to fourth thoracic **ganglia** of the **sympathetic trunk**. Each vagus contains sensory afferents from lungs and airways, parasympathetic bronchoconstrictor and secretomotor efferents, and non-cholinergic non-adrenergic nerves (NANC). Sympathetic noradrenergic fibres supplying airway smooth are sparse in humans, and the β_2-adrenergic receptors are stimulated by circulating catecholamines from the adrenal glands (Chapter 7).

Each lung is lined by a thin membrane, the **visceral pleura**, which is continuous with the **parietal pleura**, lining the chest wall, diaphragm, pericardium and mediastinum. The space between the parietal and visceral layers is tiny in health and lubricated with pleural fluid. The right and left pleural cavities are separate and each extends as the **costodiaphragmatic recess** below the lungs even during full inspiration. The parietal pleura is segmentally innervated by **intercostal nerves** and by the **phrenic nerve**, and so pain from pleural inflammation (**pleurisy**) is often referred to the chest wall or shoulder-tip. The visceral pleura lacks sensory innervation.

Lymph channels are absent in alveolar walls, but accompany small blood vessels conveying lymph towards the hilar **bronchopulmonary nodes** and from there to **tracheobronchial nodes** at the tracheal bifurcation. Some lymph from the lower lobe drains to the **posterior mediastinal nodes**.

The **upper respiratory tract** consists of the nose, pharynx and larynx. The **lower respiratory tract** (Fig. 1b) starts with the trachea at the lower border of the **cricoid cartilage**, level with the sixth cervical vertebra (C6). It bifurcates into **right** and **left main bronchi** at the level of the **sternal angle** and T4/5 (lower when upright and in inspiration). The right main bronchus is wider, shorter and more vertical than the left, so inhaled foreign bodies enter it more easily.

Airways

The airways divide repeatedly, with each successive **generation** approximately doubling in number. The **trachea** and **main bronchi** have U-shaped cartilage, linked posteriorly by smooth muscle. Lobar bronchi supply the three right and two left lung lobes and divide to give **segmental bronchi** (generations 3 and 4). The total cross-sectional area of each generation is minimum here, after which it rises rapidly, as increased numbers more than make up for their reduced size. Generations 5–11 are small bronchi, the smallest being 1 mm in diameter. The lobar, segmental and small bronchi are supported by irregular plates of cartilage, with bronchial smooth muscle forming helical bands. **Bronchioles** start at about generation 12 and from this point onwards cartilage is absent. These airways are embedded in lung tissue, which holds them open like tent guy ropes. The **terminal bronchioles** (generation 16) lead to **respiratory bronchioles**, the first generation to have alveoli (Chapter 5) in their walls. These lead to **alveolar ducts** and **alveolar sacs** (generation 23), whose walls are entirely composed of **alveoli**.

The bronchi and airways down to the terminal bronchioles receive nutrition from the **bronchial arteries** arising from the descending aorta. The respiratory bronchioles, alveolar ducts and sacs are supplied by the **pulmonary circulation** (Chapter 13).

The airways from trachea to respiratory bronchioles are lined with **ciliated columnar epithelial cells**. **Goblet cells** and **submucosal glands** secrete **mucus**. Synchronous beating of cilia moves the mucus and associated debris to the mouth (**mucociliary clearance**) (Chapters 18). Epithelial cells forming the walls of alveoli and alveolar ducts are unciliated, and largely very thin **type I alveolar pneumocytes** (alveolar cells, *squamous epithelium*). These form the gas exchange surface with the capillary endothelium (**alveolar–capillary membrane**). The **type II pneumocytes** make up only a small proportion of the alveolar surface area and are mostly found at the junction between alveoli. They are stem cells, which can divide following lung damage. They secrete **surfactant**, which reduces surface tension and has a role in lung immunity (Chapter 6 and 18). A similar substance is produced by the non-ciliated Clara cells found in the bronchiolar epithelium close to their junction with alveoli.

Dead space

The upper respiratory tract and airways as far as the terminal bronchioles do not take part in gas exchange. These **conducting airways** form the **anatomical dead space** whose volume (V_D) is normally about 150 mL. These airways have an air-conditioning function, warming, filtering and humidifying inspired air.

Alveoli that have lost their blood supply– for example because of a **pulmonary embolus** – no longer take part in gas exchange and form **alveolar dead space**. The sum of the anatomical and alveolar dead space is known as the **physiological dead space**, ventilation of which is wasted in terms of gas exchange. In health, all alveoli take part in gas exchange, so physiological dead space equals anatomical dead space.

The volume of a breath or **tidal volume** (V_T) is about 500 mL at rest. Resting **respiratory frequency** (f) is about 15 breaths/min, so the volume entering the lungs each minute, the **minute ventilation** ($\dot{V}$), is about 7500 mL/min (= 500 × 15) at rest. **Alveolar ventilation** ($\dot{V}_A$) is the volume taking part in gas exchange each minute. At rest, with a dead-space volume of 150 mL, alveolar ventilation is about 5250 mL/min (= (500 − 150) × 15).

The **Bohr method** for measuring anatomical dead space is based on the principle that the degree to which dead-space gas (0% CO_2) dilutes alveolar gas (~5% CO_2) to give mixed expired gas (~3.5%) depends on its volume (Fig. 1c). **Alveolar gas** can be sampled at the end of the breath as **end-tidal gas**. The Bohr equation can be modified to measure physiological dead space by using arterial P_{CO_2} to estimate the CO_2 in the gas-exchanging or **ideal alveoli**.

The thoracic cage and respiratory muscles

2

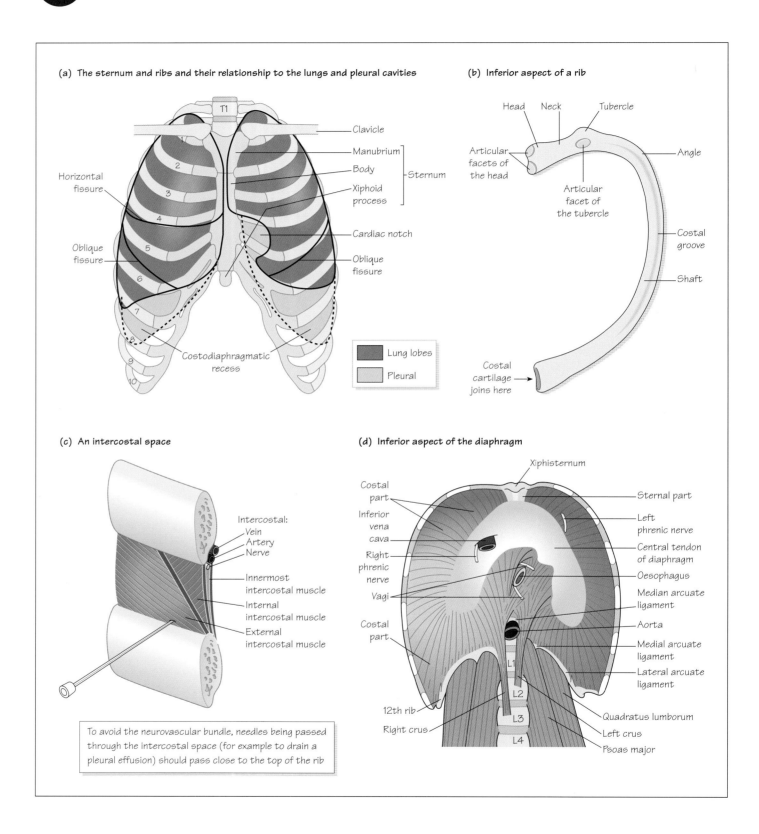

(a) The sternum and ribs and their relationship to the lungs and pleural cavities

- T1
- Clavicle
- Manubrium
- Body
- Xiphoid process
- Sternum
- Horizontal fissure
- Oblique fissure
- Cardiac notch
- Oblique fissure
- Costodiaphragmatic recess
- Lung lobes
- Pleural

(b) Inferior aspect of a rib

- Head
- Neck
- Tubercle
- Articular facets of the head
- Articular facet of the tubercle
- Angle
- Costal groove
- Shaft
- Costal cartilage joins here

(c) An intercostal space

- Intercostal:
  - Vein
  - Artery
  - Nerve
- Innermost intercostal muscle
- Internal intercostal muscle
- External intercostal muscle

To avoid the neurovascular bundle, needles being passed through the intercostal space (for example to drain a pleural effusion) should pass close to the top of the rib

(d) Inferior aspect of the diaphragm

- Xiphisternum
- Costal part
- Inferior vena cava
- Right phrenic nerve
- Vagi
- Costal part
- 12th rib
- Right crus
- Sternal part
- Left phrenic nerve
- Central tendon of diaphragm
- Oesophagus
- Median arcuate ligament
- Aorta
- Medial arcuate ligament
- Lateral arcuate ligament
- Quadratus lumborum
- Left crus
- Psoas major
- L1
- L2
- L3
- L4

 The Respiratory System at a Glance, 3e. By J.P.T. Ward, J. Ward, R.M. Leach. Published 2010 Blackwell Publishing Ltd.

Thoracic cage

The **thoracic cage** is composed of the **sternum**, **ribs**, **intercostal spaces** and **thoracic vertebral column**, with the **diaphragm** dividing the thorax from the abdomen.

The sternum

The dagger-shaped **sternum** has three parts. The **manubrium**, with which the first and upper parts of the second costal cartilage and the clavicle articulate (Fig. 2a), lies at the level of the third and fourth thoracic vertebrae (see Fig. 1b). The lower parts of the second and third to seventh ribs articulate with the **body of the sternum** (level with T5–T8). The angle between the manubrium and body at the cartilaginous **manubriosternal joint** forms the **sternal angle (angle of Louis)**, and this is a useful anatomical reference point. The small **xiphoid process** (xiphisternum) usually remains cartilaginous well into adult life.

The ribs and intercostal space

The first 7 (**true** or **vertebrosternal**) of the 12 pairs of ribs are connected to the sternum by their costal cartilages. The hyaline cartilages of the eighth, ninth and tenth (false or **vertebrochondral**) ribs articulate with the cartilage above, and the eleventh and twelfth are free (**floating** or **vertebral ribs**). A typical rib (Fig. 2b) has a **head** with two **facets** for articulation with the corresponding vertebra, the intervertebral disc and the vertebra above. The rib also articulates at the **tubercle** with the transverse process of the corresponding vertebra. The two articular regions act like a hinge, forcing the rib to move through an axis passing through these areas. The flattened shaft of the rib is weakest at the **angle of the rib** and this is where it tends to fracture in an adult. The upper two ribs, protected by the clavicle and the two floating ribs, are least likely to fracture. There is a cervical rib attached to the transverse process of C7 in 0.5% of people, and the presence of this rib may cause paraesthesiae or vascular problems, due to pressure on the brachial plexus or subclavian artery.

Intercostal spaces contain **external intercostal muscles** whose fibres pass downwards and forwards between the ribs, **internal intercostal muscles** whose fibres pass downwards and backwards and an incomplete **innermost intercostal layer** (Fig. 2c). They are innervated by **intercostal nerves**, which are the anterior primary rami of **thoracic nerves**. **Intercostal veins**, **arteries** and **nerves** lie in grooves on the undersurface of the corresponding rib, with the vein above, artery in the middle and nerve below.

The diaphragm

The dome-shaped **diaphragm** (Fig. 2d) separates the thorax and abdomen and consists of a muscular peripheral part and a **central tendon**, which is partly fused with the pericardium. The muscular diaphragm takes its origin from the vertebrae and arcuate ligaments, the rib cage and the sternum. The **right crus** arises from the upper three lumbar vertebrae and the **left crus** from the upper two lumbar vertebrae. Their fibrous medial borders form the **median arcuate ligament** over the front of the aorta. The **medial** and **lateral arcuate ligaments** are thickenings of the fascia overlying the **psoas major** and **quadratus lumborum**, respectively. The costal part of the diaphragm is attached to the inner aspects of the seventh to twelfth ribs and costal cartilages.

The sternal part originates as two slips from the back of the xiphisternum. The **phrenic nerves (C3, 4, 5)** supply motor fibres. Sensory innervation of the central diaphragm also runs in the phrenic, and pain from irritation of the diaphragm is often referred to the corresponding dermatome for C4, the shoulder-tip. The lower intercostal nerves supply sensory fibres to the peripheral diaphragm. The aorta, thoracic duct and azygos vein pass through the diaphragm at the aortic opening at the level of T12. The oesophagus, branches of the left gastric artery and vein and both vagi pass through the oesophageal opening at the level of T10, and the inferior vena cava and right phrenic nerve pass through an opening at the level of T8.

Muscles of respiration

All inspiratory muscles act to increase thoracic volume, causing intrapleural and alveolar pressure to fall to create an alveolar–mouth pressure gradient, drawing air into the lungs. The expanded chest wall and lungs will recoil by themselves and quiet breathing uses no expiratory muscles.

The main inspiratory muscle, the **diaphragm**, moves down when it contracts, by about 1.5 cm during quiet breathing and 6–7 cm during deep breathing. During quiet breathing, the first rib remains fairly still and the **intercostal muscles** elevate and evert the succeeding ribs. The intercostal muscles also stiffen the intercostal spaces preventing them from being sucked in during inspiration. The **scalene muscles**, which insert into the first two ribs, are also active in normal inspiration. Raising the upper ribs pushes the sternum forward (the **pump action**) increasing the anterior–posterior diameter of the chest, and as the sloping lower ribs rise, they move out (the **bucket-handle action**) and the transverse diameter of the chest wall increases.

In quiet breathing in adults, ventilation is largely diaphragmatic. As the diaphragm contracts, it squashes the abdominal contents and raises intra-abdominal pressure, pushing out the abdominal wall and lower ribs. Consequently, in normal breathing the chest wall and the abdominal wall move out together during inspiration. If the diaphragm is paralysed, increased chest volume is produced entirely by raising the ribs, and as intrathoracic pressure falls in inspiration, the flaccid diaphragm is sucked into the chest and the abdomen moves in. This out-of-phase movement of the chest and abdominal walls is known as **paradoxical breathing**. In a high cervical cord transection, all respiratory muscles are paralysed, but when the damage is below the phrenic nerve roots (C3, 4, 5) breathing continues via the diaphragm alone. In the newborn, ribs are horizontal, so rib movements cannot increase the volume of the chest and breathing is entirely by the up-and-down action of the diaphragm or so-called **abdominal breathing**. As the ribs become more oblique with increasing age, there is an increased contribution of **thoracic breathing**.

When ventilation or resistance to breathing is increased, **accessory inspiratory muscles** aid inspiration. These include the **scalene muscles**, **sternomastoids** and **serratus anterior**. If the arms are fixed by grasping the edge of a table, contraction of the **pectoralis major**, which normally adducts the arm, helps expand the chest. When ventilation exceeds about 40 L/min, there is activation of expiratory muscles, especially **abdominal muscles (rectus abdominis**, **external** and **internal oblique)**, which speeds up recoil of the diaphragm by raising intra-abdominal pressure.

3 Pressures and volumes during normal breathing

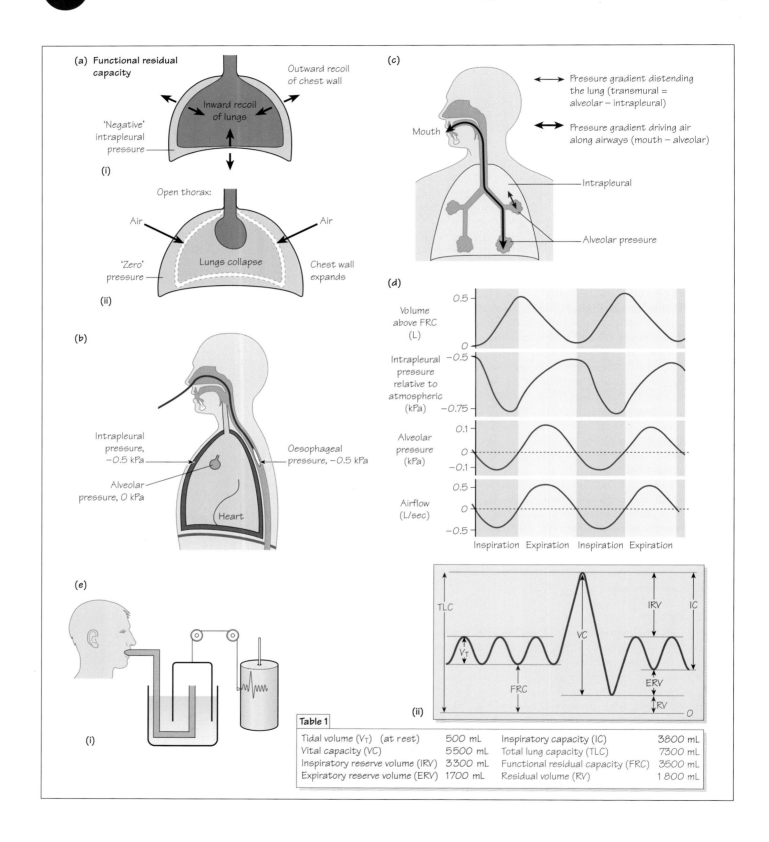

(a) Functional residual capacity

Outward recoil of chest wall

Inward recoil of lungs

'Negative' intrapleural pressure

(i)

Open thorax:

Air

Air

'Zero' pressure

Lungs collapse

Chest wall expands

(ii)

(b)

Intrapleural pressure, −0.5 kPa

Oesophageal pressure, −0.5 kPa

Alveolar pressure, 0 kPa

Heart

(c)

Pressure gradient distending the lung (transmural = alveolar − intrapleural)

Pressure gradient driving air along airways (mouth − alveolar)

Mouth

Intrapleural

Alveolar pressure

(d)

Volume above FRC (L)

Intrapleural pressure relative to atmospheric (kPa)

Alveolar pressure (kPa)

Airflow (L/sec)

Inspiration Expiration Inspiration Expiration

(e)

(i)

(ii)

TLC   IRV   IC

VC

V_T

FRC

ERV

RV

0

Table 1

Tidal volume (V_T) (at rest)	500 mL	Inspiratory capacity (IC)	3800 mL
Vital capacity (VC)	5500 mL	Total lung capacity (TLC)	7300 mL
Inspiratory reserve volume (IRV)	3300 mL	Functional residual capacity (FRC)	3500 mL
Expiratory reserve volume (ERV)	1700 mL	Residual volume (RV)	1800 mL

Functional residual capacity

The volume left in the lungs at the end of a normal breath is known as the **functional residual capacity (FRC)**. At FRC, the respiratory muscles are relaxed and its volume is determined by the elastic properties of the lungs and chest wall.

The lungs are elastic bodies whose resting volume when removed from the body is very small. The natural resting position of the chest wall, seen when the chest is opened surgically, is about 1 L larger than at the end of a normal breath.

In the living respiratory system, the lungs are sealed within the chest wall. Between these two elastic structures is the **intrapleural space**, which contains only a few millilitres of fluid. When the respiratory muscles are relaxed, the lungs and chest wall recoil in opposite directions, creating a subatmospheric ('negative') pressure in the space between them, and this tends to oppose the recoil of both the lungs and the chest wall. FRC occurs when the **outward recoil** of the chest wall exactly balances the **inward recoil** of the lungs (Fig. 3a). When the chest is opened, air enters the intrapleural space, the pressure becomes atmospheric and nothing opposes the recoil of the lungs and chest wall. The lungs shrink to a small volume and the chest wall springs out.

If the elastic recoil of either the lungs or the chest wall is abnormally large or small, FRC will be abnormal. In lung fibrosis, the lungs are stiff and have increased elastic recoil, so the balance point, and hence FRC, occurs at a small lung volume. In emphysema, there is loss of alveolar tissue and with it, loss of elastic recoil. When the respiratory muscles are relaxed, the reduced elastic recoil of the lungs offers less opposition to the outward recoil of the chest wall and FRC is increased (the **barrel chest** of emphysema). Increased FRC can also occur because of 'air trapping' (see Chapter 7).

Intrapleural pressure

The space between the **visceral pleura** lining the lungs and the **parietal pleura** lining the chest wall is so small that measuring **intrapleural pressure** with a needle risks puncturing the lung. Intrapleural pressure can be indirectly assessed from **oesophageal pressure** (Fig. 3b). The oesophagus is normally closed at the top and bottom except during swallowing and in the upright subject the oesophageal pressure is the same as in the neighbouring intrapleural space. The subject swallows either a miniaturized pressure transducer or a balloon containing a little air connected by a tube to an external manometer. Gravity affects the fluid-lined intrapleural space, and at FRC in an upright subject, the intrapleural pressure at the apex of the lungs is about −0.5 kPa (−5 cmH₂O) and about −0.2 kPa (−2 cmH₂O) at the bottom.

Pressures, flow and volume during a normal breathing cycle

During inspiration, the chest wall is expanded and intrapleural pressure falls. This increases the pressure gradient between the intrapleural space and alveoli (Fig. 3c), stretching the lungs. The alveoli expand and **alveolar pressure** falls, creating a pressure gradient between the mouth and alveoli, causing air to flow into the lungs. The airflow profile (Fig. 3d) closely follows that of alveolar pressure. During expiration, both intrapleural pressure and alveolar pressure rise. In quiet breathing, intrapleural pressure remains negative for the whole respiratory cycle, whereas alveolar pressure is negative during inspiration and positive during expiration. Alveolar pressure is always higher than intrapleural because of the recoil of the lung. It is zero at the end of both inspiration and expiration, and airflow ceases momentarily. When ventilation is increased, the changes of intrapleural and alveolar pressure are greater and in expiration intrapleural pressure may rise above atmospheric pressure. In forced expiration, coughing or sneezing, intrapleural pressure may rise to +8 kPa (+60 mmHg) or more.

Lung volumes

If a subject breathes in and out of a **simple water-filled spirometer** (Fig. 3e(i)), the drum falls and rises and the pen, attached by a pulley system, produces a trace (Fig. 3e(ii)) which illustrates the important lung volumes. Conventionally, volumes composed of two or more volumes are known as 'capacities', whereas those that cannot be subdivided are known as 'volumes'. The volume breathed in (or out) is known as the **tidal volume**, and the trace shows several **resting tidal volumes**, which are typically about 500 mL. At the end of a normal quiet inspiration, the subject could breathe in more and this is the **inspiratory reserve volume (IRV)**. Similarly, the volume that he or she could exhale after a normal expiration is the **expiratory reserve volume (ERV)**. For the fourth breath, the subject breathes in and out as fully as possible. This maximum tidal volume is the **vital capacity ($VC = V_T + IRV + ERV$)**. At the end of a maximal breath out, the volume remaining in the lungs is the **residual volume**. FRC and **total lung capacity** are the volumes in the lungs at the end of a normal expiration and after a maximal breath in, respectively. Possible values for a man are given in Table 1. Although a zero volume line is shown (Fig. 3e(ii)), it is not possible to know where this actually is on a trace, because the subject cannot empty the lungs into the drum. For this reason, although illustrated in Fig. 3e(ii), volumes shown in red in Table 1 cannot be measured from a simple spirometer trace. They can be measured using **helium dilution** or **body plethysmography** (Chapter 20). The range of normal lung volumes is large and an individual's volumes must be assessed with the aid of **nomograms** that give the predicted value of each volume for the subject's age, sex and height.

4 Gas laws

(a) Altitude, barometric pressure, O_2 fraction and PO_2

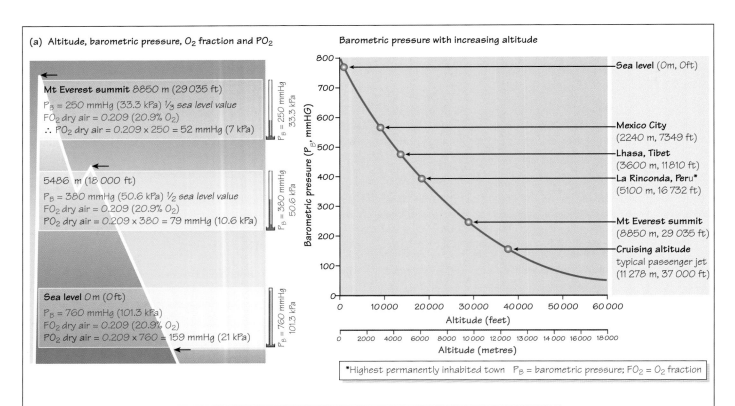

Mt Everest summit *8850 m (29 035 ft)*
P_B = 250 mmHg (33.3 kPa) ⅓ sea level value
FO_2 dry air = 0.209 (20.9% O_2)
∴ PO_2 dry air = 0.209 × 250 = 52 mmHg (7 kPa)

P_B = 250 mmHg 33.3 kPa

5486 m (18 000 ft)
P_B = 380 mmHg (50.6 kPa) ½ sea level value
FO_2 dry air = 0.209 (20.9% O_2)
PO_2 dry air = 0.209 × 380 = 79 mmHg (10.6 kPa)

P_B = 380 mmHg 50.6 kPa

Sea level *0 m (0 ft)*
P_B = 760 mmHg (101.3 kPa)
FO_2 dry air = 0.209 (20.9% O_2)
PO_2 dry air = 0.209 × 760 = 159 mmHg (21 kPa)

P_B = 760 mmHg 101.3 kPa

Barometric pressure with increasing altitude

Barometric pressure (P_B, mmHG)

- Sea level (0 m, 0 ft)
- Mexico City (2240 m, 7349 ft)
- Lhasa, Tibet (3600 m, 11810 ft)
- La Rinconda, Peru* (5100 m, 16 732 ft)
- Mt Everest summit (8850 m, 29 035 ft)
- Cruising altitude typical passenger jet (11 278 m, 37 000 ft)

Altitude (feet)

Altitude (metres)

*Highest permanently inhabited town P_B = barometric pressure; FO_2 = O_2 fraction

(b) Correction factors for gas volumes

$$\text{Volume}_{(BTPS)} = \text{volume}_{(ATPS)} \left(\frac{273 + 37}{273 + t^\circ C}\right)\left(\frac{P_B - P_{H_2O}}{P_B - 6.3^*}\right) \quad \text{*47 if } P_B \text{ and } P_{H_2O} \text{ are in mmHg}$$

$$\text{Volume}_{(STPD)} = \text{volume}_{(ATPS)} \left(\frac{273}{273 + t^\circ C}\right)\left(\frac{P_B - P_{H_2O}}{101^*}\right) \quad \text{*760 if } P_B \text{ and } P_{H_2O} \text{ are in mmHg}$$

(c) Partial pressure of a gas in a liquid

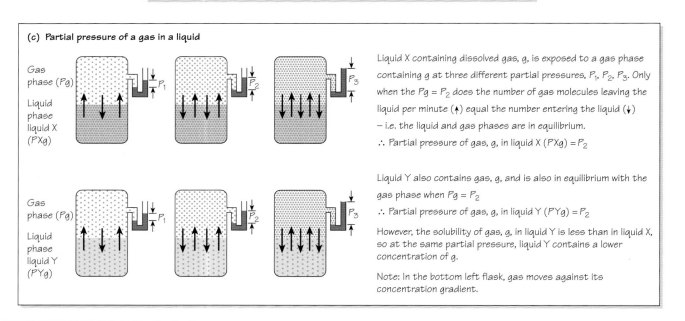

Gas phase (Pg)

Liquid phase liquid X (PXg)

P_1 P_2 P_3

Liquid X containing dissolved gas, g, is exposed to a gas phase containing g at three different partial pressures, P_1, P_2, P_3. Only when the $Pg = P_2$ does the number of gas molecules leaving the liquid per minute (↑) equal the number entering the liquid (↓) – i.e. the liquid and gas phases are in equilibrium.

∴ Partial pressure of gas, g, in liquid X (PXg) = P_2

Gas phase (Pg)

Liquid phase liquid Y (PYg)

P_1 P_2 P_3

Liquid Y also contains gas, g, and is also in equilibrium with the gas phase when $Pg = P_2$

∴ Partial pressure of gas, g, in liquid Y (PYg) = P_2

However, the solubility of gas, g, in liquid Y is less than in liquid X, so at the same partial pressure, liquid Y contains a lower concentration of g.

Note: In the bottom left flask, gas moves against its concentration gradient.

To understand the processes involved in respiration and how valid measurements are made, it is important to understand the behaviour of gases in both gas mixtures and liquids.

Fractional concentration and partial pressure of gases in a gas mixture

Dalton's law states that when two or more gases, which do not react chemically, are present in the same container, the total pressure is the sum of the partial pressures (the pressure that each gas would exert if isolated in the container).

The total pressure exerted by the atmosphere was traditionally measured by inverting a long mercury-filled glass tube over a mercury reservoir. At sea level, the height of the column supported is normally about 760 mm, so barometric pressure is 760 mmHg (1 mmHg $\cong$ 1 torr), which in SI units is about 101 kPa (1 kPa = 7.50 mmHg). Dried air contains approximately 21% oxygen (i.e. oxygen fraction (FO_2) $\approx$0.21). The remaining gases are nitrogen, 78.1%, and inert gases such as argon and helium, 0.9%, although for convenience these physiologically inert gases are often pooled as 'nitrogen, 79%'. Air is considered to be CO_2-free, as the amount present (0.04%) is very small. According to Dalton's law:

Dry partial pressure oxygen in inspired air (P_{IO_2})
= oxygen fraction (F_{O_2}) × total barometric pressure (P_B)
= 0.21 × 101 (760) = 21.2 kPa (159 mmHg)

At **altitude**, the oxygen fraction of air is unaltered, but barometric pressure is reduced, being about 33.6 kPa (252 mmHg) on the top of Everest (Fig. 4a).

Water vapour pressure

Air contains variable amounts of water vapour, depending on the water it has been exposed to and the temperature. The maximum or **saturated water vapour pressure** is higher in warm than in cool air: at 20°C, it is 2.33 kPa (17.5 mmHg), whereas at body temperature (37°C), it is 6.3 kPa (47 mmHg). The **relative humidity** (actual/saturated water vapour pressure × 100%) of inspired air varies with the weather; if it is 40% at 20°C, water vapour pressure will be 0.9 kPa (7 mmHg). The presence of water vapour means that ambient FO_2 and FN_2 are usually a little lower than the dry fractions given above. Air passing down the airways quickly reaches body temperature (37°C) and 100% saturation. Total pressure remains close to barometric, so the added water vapour causes significant dilution of the other gases. The available pressure for the other gases is therefore P_B −6.3 kPa (P_B −47 mmHg).

The **partial pressure of moist inspired oxygen (P_{IO_2})** = 0.21×
(P_B − saturated vapour pressure at 37°C)

Moistened inspired P_{IO_2} is always 1.3 kPa (= 0.21 × 6.1) or 10 mmHg less than dry P_{O_2}. Note that this has a proportionally greater effect on P_{IO_2} at high altitude than at sea level. If dry air is saturated with water at 37°C, at sea level P_{IO_2} falls by 6% from 21.2 to 19.9 kPa (159–149 mmHg); on the summit of Everest, P_{IO_2} falls from 7.0 to 5.7 kPa (52–42 mmHg), a 19% reduction.

The effect of pressure and temperature on gas volumes

The inverse relationship between the volume of a perfect gas and its pressure, described by **Boyle's law** (P $\propto$ 1/V), and the direct relationship between volume and absolute temperature (= 273 + °C), described by **Charles' law** (V $\propto$ T), are important when measuring gas volumes. Expired gas collected in a bag or spirometer will shrink, both because of the direct effect of falling temperature (Charles' law) and because water vapour condenses as temperature falls. To enable valid comparisons, volumes at **ambient temperature and pressure saturated with water (ATPS)** are corrected to those they would occupy under standard conditions. For measurements of lung volumes, this is to **body temperature and pressure saturated with water (BTPS)**. For O_2 consumption or CO_2 production, **standard temperature and pressure dry (STPD)** (0°C, 101.3 kPa (760 mmHg), $P_{H_2O} = 0$) are usually used, so that each litre contains the same number of molecules (1 mole $\approx$ 22.4 L).

Boyle's law, Charles' law and the reduction of saturated vapour pressure with temperature are combined in the equations for correcting volumes given in Fig. 4b.

Gases dissolved in liquids

If a gas is exposed to a liquid to which it does not react, gas particles will move into the liquid. **Henry's law** states that the number of molecules dissolving in the liquid is directly proportional to the partial pressure at the surface of the gas.

The constant of proportionality is the solubility of the gas in the liquid, and it is affected by the gas, the liquid and the temperature, tending to fall as temperature rises.

Content of dissolved gas X in a liquid Y = solubility of X in Y× partial pressure of X at surface

The **partial pressure of a gas in a liquid** or **gas tension** is a more difficult concept than that of partial pressure in a gas phase, where we can visualize the pressure of the molecules holding up a column of mercury. The molecules of the gas in the liquid phase will move about in the liquid and have a tendency to escape from the surface, which can be opposed by molecules of the same gas in a gas phase in contact with the liquid (Fig. 4c). If the partial pressure of the gas in the gas phase is altered until there is no net movement of gas between the gas phase and the liquid phase, the gas and liquid are said to be in equilibrium. By definition, the partial pressure of a gas in a liquid is equal to the partial pressure of that gas in a gas phase with which it is in equilibrium. Partial pressure gradient (not concentration gradient) always determines the direction of movement between phases such as a gas and liquid phase.

Note on time derivative symbols

Standard symbols used in respiratory physiology are given in Units and Symbols on page 7. Time derivatives are properly denoted by a dot over the symbol (e.g. $\dot{V}_A$, alveolar ventilation in L/min, see Units and Symbols on page 7). However, for terms such as the ventilation–perfusion ratio (V_A/Q) the dots are often omitted, and this convention is followed throughout this book.

5 Diffusion

(a) The alveolar–capillary membrane

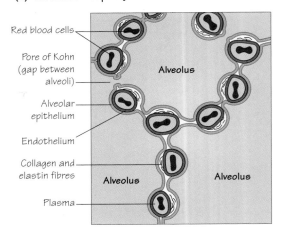

Red blood cells

Pore of Kohn (gap between alveoli)

Alveolar epithelium

Endothelium

Collagen and elastin fibres

Plasma

Alveolus

Alveolus

Alveolus

(b) Transfer of gases across alveolar–capillary membrane

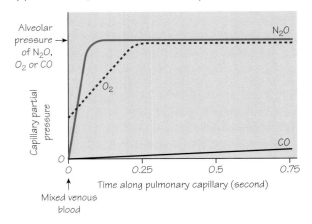

(c) Diffusion through a sheet of tissue

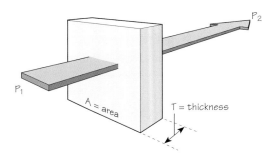

P_2

P_1

A = area

T = thickness

(e) The oxygen cascade: oxygen tension from ambient air to mitochondria

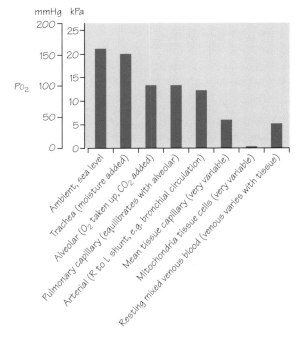

(d) The diffusion path through the alveolar–capillary membrane

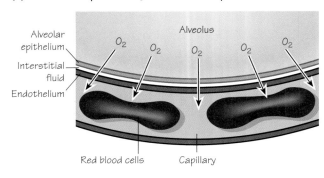

Alveolar epithelium

Interstitial fluid

Endothelium

Alveolus

O_2 O_2 O_2 O_2 O_2

Red blood cells   Capillary

Oxygen and carbon dioxide are transported in the body by a mixture of **bulk flow** and **diffusion**. Bulk flow, generated by differences in total fluid pressure, is important in most of the airways and in transporting blood containing these gases between pulmonary and tissue capillaries. Diffusion, driven by partial pressure differences, is important in the last few millimetres of the airways, across the alveolar–capillary membrane and between tissue capillaries and mitochondria.

The alveolar–capillary membrane (Fig. 5a)

Adult male lungs contain about 300 million alveoli, approximately 0.2 mm in diameter. Between neighbouring alveoli are two layers of **alveolar epithelium** each resting on a basement membrane, enclosing the interstitial space, containing **pulmonary capillaries**, **elastin** and **collagen fibres**. The **alveolar epithelium** and **capillary endothelium** form the **alveolar–capillary membrane**, through which gases diffuse. It is very thin (<0.4 μm), except where collagen and elastin fibres are concentrated, with a total surface area of about 85 m^2. There are two types of alveolar epithelial cells. **Type I pneumocytes** line the alveoli and are relatively devoid of organelles. The round **type II pneumocytes** have large nuclei, microvilli and contain striated osmiophilic lamellar bodies storing surfactant, an important component of alveolar lining fluid (Chapter 6).

Diffusion and perfusion limitation (Fig. 5b)

If gas containing the poorly soluble gas nitrous oxide (N_2O) is inhaled, pulmonary capillary P_{N_2O} rises and quickly equilibrates with alveolar P_{N_2O}. With no alveolar–capillary partial pressure gradient remaining, diffusion ceases along the rest of the pulmonary capillary and uptake can only be increased by increasing pulmonary capillary blood flow. N_2O uptake is said to be **perfusion-limited**. In contrast, when breathing a carbon monoxide (CO) containing mixture, the CO combines so avidly with haemoglobin that pulmonary capillary P_{CO} rises little. The pressure gradient driving diffusion is preserved along the capillary, and CO uptake would not be increased by increased perfusion. Improved ease of diffusion, with reduced thickness or increased area of the alveolar–capillary membrane, would increase CO uptake. CO transfer is **diffusion-limited**. Oxygen transfer lies between these two extremes, but is normally perfusion-limited.

Factors affecting diffusion across a membrane (Fick and Graham's laws)

For a sheet of tissue of area A and thickness T through which gas g is passing (Fig. 5c):

Rate of transfer of gas, $g \propto \dfrac{A}{T}(P_1 - P_2)$

The constant of proportionality

$$= \frac{\text{Solubility of the gas in the membrane(s)}}{\sqrt{\text{Molecular weight of the gas}}}$$

Although the molecular weight of CO_2 is about 1.4 times that of O_2, it is about 20 times more soluble, and so diffuses more easily.

For the alveolar–capillary membrane, the pressure gradient driving diffusion is alveolar (P_A) minus mean pulmonary capillary ($P_{\bar{C}}$). The constants (s, mw, A and T) can be combined to give a single constant, the **diffusing capacity** ($D_L g$) of the lungs for gas, g:

Rate of transfer of gas, $g = D_L g(P_A - P_{\bar{C}})$

Oxygen diffusing capacity, $D_L O_2$

$$= \frac{\text{Oxygen uptake from the lungs } (\dot{V}_{O_2})}{P_A O_2 - P_{\bar{C}} O_2}$$

Although measurement of $D_L O_2$ is desirable, it is not possible because mean capillary P_{O_2} ($P_{\bar{C}} O_2$) cannot be measured. CO diffuses through the same pathway as O_2, and its rate of diffusion is affected by the same factors that affect oxygen transfer. However, unlike $D_L O_2$, $D_L CO$ is measurable. Once CO arrives in the pulmonary capillary blood, it too combines with haemoglobin. Haemoglobin has approximately 240 times the affinity for CO than it does for O_2, and consequently as CO is transferred, almost all of it enters chemical combination and the mean pulmonary capillary P_{CO} can be assumed to be zero.

This simplifies the equation to:

$$D_L CO = \frac{\text{Carbon monoxide uptake from the lungs } (\dot{V}_{CO})}{P_A CO}$$

Several methods are used for measuring $D_L CO$, but all involve breathing a low level of CO (e.g. 0.3%). By sampling exhaled gas, CO uptake and mean alveolar P_{CO} can be calculated. The normal value depends on the method used, but is about 15–30 mL/min per mmHg (112–225 mL/min per kPa). A tracer gas, such as helium, is included in the gas mixture so that alveolar volume can also be measured (see Chapter 20). $D_L CO$ is divided by alveolar volume to give an index (K_{CO}) that corrects for different lung volumes. As both $D_L O_2$ and $D_L CO$ are affected by the rate of gas combination with haemoglobin in addition to factors affecting diffusion, the alternative term, transfer factor ($T_L O_2$ and $T_L CO$), is more commonly used in Europe.

Factors affecting $D_L CO$ ($T_L CO$)

$D_L CO$ is lowered by reduced alveolar–capillary membrane area in emphysema, pulmonary emboli or lung resection and by increased thickness in pulmonary oedema. In pulmonary fibrosis the alveolar–capillary membrane is both thickened and reduced in area giving a low $D_L CO$ with a low but less affected K_{CO}. Increased pulmonary blood volume in exercise increases the effective area increasing $D_L CO$. $D_L CO$ is increased with polycythaemia and reduced in anaemia. $D_L CO$ is therefore non-specific, but it is sensitive and may reveal abnormalities when other lung function tests are normal. Hypoventilation does not affect $D_L CO$ because the reduced CO uptake is caused by reduced $P_A CO$.

The oxygen cascade (Fig. 5e) shows how P_{O_2} falls between air and mitochondria. Mitochondrial oxidative phosphorylation will cease when P_{O_2} falls below 1 mmHg (0.13 kPa), and this ultimately limits the capillary P_{O_2} that can be tolerated and therefore the amount of oxygen that can be removed as blood passes through the tissues. Capillary P_{O_2} must remain high enough to drive diffusion to cells at a rate sufficient to match oxygen consumption and maintain mitochondrial P_{O_2} above this critical level.

6 Lung mechanics: elastic forces

(a) Static pressure–volume loop

Volume % TLC

100

50 — FRC

RV

0

C_L = slope ΔV/ΔP

ΔV

ΔP

10   20   cmH₂O

0   1   2   kPa

Transmural pressure (= – intrapleural pressure since measurements taken at zero airflow)

RV = Residual volume   FRC = Functional residual capacity
TLC = Total lung capacity C_L = Lung compliance

(b) Dynamic pressure–volume loop

If intrapleural pressure and volume are recorded continuously (lower panel), a pressure–volume loop (upper panel) can be constructed from pairs of simultaneous measurements of volume, e.g. (b) with pressure (b'). Alternatively the pressure and volume signals can be fed into an X-Y plotter.

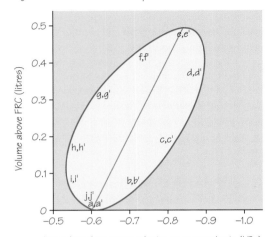

Intrapleural pressure relative to atmospheric (kPa)

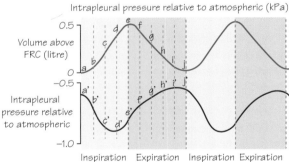

Inspiration Expiration Inspiration Expiration

(c) Surface tension

R

Pressure above ambient = P

Laplace's equation

$$P = \frac{2T}{R}$$

T = Surface tension

P_1

P_2

$P_1 > P_2$

∴ When tap is opened the small bubble empties into the large

(d) Effect of surface area

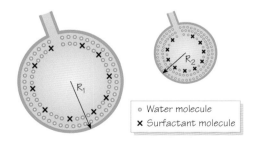

○ Water molecule
✕ Surfactant molecule

$R_2 < R_1$ but $T_2 < T_1$ because surface concentration of surfactant is higher when the alveolus is small
The fall in R is more than offset by the fall in T,
∴ since $P = \dfrac{2T}{R}$, P does not rise, but falls as the alveolus shrinks

To breathe in, the inspiratory muscles must contract to overcome the impedance offered by the lungs and chest wall. This is mainly in the form of frictional **airway resistance** (Chapter 7) and **elastic resistance** to stretching of the lung and chest wall tissues and the fluid lining the alveoli.

Assessing the stiffness of the lungs: lung compliance

The 'stretchiness' of the lung is usually assessed as lung compliance (C_L), which is the change in lung volume per unit change in distending pressure ($C_L = \Delta V/\Delta P$). The distending pressure, P, is the pressure difference across the lung, which equals alveolar–intrapleural pressure.

Intrapleural pressure can be assessed by measuring oesophageal pressure (Chapter 3). Alveolar pressure cannot easily be measured directly, but when no air is flowing, alveolar pressure must equal mouth pressure (i.e. zero). The transmural pressure, P, is then equal to intrapleural pressure. The subject breathes in steps and measurements are taken while the breath is held and plotted as a **static pressure–volume (P–V) curve** (Fig. 6a). The curve flattens as the lung volume approaches total lung capacity (TLC). The inspiratory curve is slightly different from the expiratory curve, and this **hysteresis** is a common property of elastic bodies. **Static lung compliance** is the slope of the steepest part of this static pressure–volume curve in the region just above functional residual capacity (FRC).

Lung compliance is normally about 1.5 L/kPa, but as with lung volumes it is affected by the subject's size, age and gender. In **restrictive disease**, such as lung fibrosis, lung compliance is low. Like a stiff spring, once stretched, fibrosed lungs have an increased tendency to shrink back to their resting position or increased **elastic recoil**. The loss of alveolar tissue in **emphysema** makes them easier to stretch and lung compliance is increased. Although safe, swallowing an oesophageal balloon is not very pleasant or convenient. Fortunately, it is often possible to deduce that a patient has stiff lungs from other measurements such as **TLC**, **FRC** (Chapters 3, 20 and 30), forced expiratory volume in 1 second (**FEV_1**) and forced vital capacity (**FVC**) (Chapter 20).

Dynamic pressure–volume loops and dynamic compliance

A **dynamic pressure–volume loop** (upper panel of Fig. 6b) is obtained from continuous measurements of intrapleural pressure and volume during a normal breathing cycle (lower panel of Fig. 6b). There are two points, at the ends of inspiration and expiration, where airflow and alveolar pressure are zero (a, a' and e, e') and the slope of the line joining these points is **dynamic compliance**. In health, its value is similar to the **static compliance**, but in some diseases it may be lower, as stiff areas may fill preferentially during normal breathing. Between the two zero flow points, the dynamic P–V loop appears fatter than the static P–V loop, as intrapleural pressure must change more to drive airflow. In fact, the area of the dynamic loop is a measure of the work done against airway resistance (Chapter 7).

The air–fluid interface lining the alveoli

During inspiration, as well as stretching the collagen and elastin fibres, the **surface tension** forces at the air–alveolar lining fluid interface must be overcome. At the surface of a bubble, the attraction of the fluid molecules for each other creates a tension, which tends to shrink the bubble (Fig. 6c). Laplace discovered that a gas bubble in a liquid would shrink until the pressure, P, within it reached a value of 2T/R, where T is a constant, the surface tension of the fluid, and R is the radius of the bubble. When a bubble has air on both sides, there are two air–fluid interfaces and P = 4T/R. The **law of Laplace** (P = 2T/R or 4T/R) predicts that, if two bubbles are made of the same fluid, the smaller bubble will have a higher pressure within it – since when the radius of curvature is small, a greater proportion of the surface tension is directed to the centre of the bubble (lower panel of Fig. 6.1c). When the two bubbles are connected, the small bubble empties into the large bubble as air flows down the pressure gradient.

The lungs are not a simple system of bubbles connected by tubes but much more complicated. In life alveoli are not spherical, they have interconnections between neighbouring alveoli and alveolar fluid may not produce a continuous lining to the alveoli. Nevertheless, the surface tension forces illustrated by this model are undoubtedly important in the lung and the presence of an air–fluid interface creates several potential problems:

1 It reduces lung compliance and the higher the surface tension the lower the compliance.

2 The alveoli and small airways would be inherently unstable, tending to collapse under surface tension forces during expiration resulting in areas of **atelectasis**.

The absence of these problems in healthy humans is thought to be partly due to the presence in the alveolar lining fluid of **surfactant**.

Surfactant

Pulmonary surfactant is a mixture of **phospholipids**, such phosphatidylcholine and proteins, produced by the **type II pneumocytes** (Chapter 5). The presence of these substances in the **alveolar lining fluid** lowers the surface tension and increases compliance. The phospholipids have a **hydrophilic** end that lies in the alveolar fluid and a **hydrophobic** end that projects into the alveolar gas, and as a result they float on the surface of the lining fluid. As an alveolus shrinks, its surface area diminishes and the surface concentration of surfactant rises (Fig. 6d). As surface tension falls with increasing surface concentration of surfactant, the increased tendency for alveoli to collapse when they shrink is offset and stability is improved. Alveolar stability is also aided by the connection and mutual pull of neighbouring alveoli, a phenomenon known as **alveolar interdependence**.

Surfactant production in the fetus gradually increases in the last third of pregnancy and may be inadequate in babies born prematurely, giving rise to the typical problems of **neonatal respiratory distress syndrome (NRDS)** – stiff lungs and areas of collapse (Chapters 16 and 17).

Surfactant proteins (e.g. SP-A, SP-B, SP-C and SP-D) contribute to the surface tension lowering actions of phospholipids, as well as having other functions such as host defence. They are probably the reason why natural surfactants have proved more effective for treating NRDS than artificial surfactant composed only of phospholipids.

(a) Laminar and turbulent flow

Laminar flow

Turbulent flow

(b) Main factors influencing bronchomotor tone

Bronchodilation

Bronchoconstriction

CO_2

NANC nerves *(inhibitory)*

β-Adrenergic agonists *(e.g. adrenaline and saltbutamol)*

Airway smooth muscle

NO and VIP

β_2-Receptor

Vagal efferents

ACh via M_3 receptors

SP and neurokinins

Synapse

NANC nerves *(excitatory)*

Histamine, Prostagladins Leukotrienes etc

Pulmonary stretch receptors *(inhibit)*

Brainstem *(Chapter 12)*

Airway irritant receptors *(activate)*

Mast cells, eosinophil *(Chapter 23)*

Vagal afferents

▼ = Receptor
Y = Nerve ending

NO = Nitric oxide
VIP = Vasoactive intestinal peptide
SP = Substance P

ACh = Acetylcholine
M3 = Muscarinic type 3 receptor

(d) Dynamic compression of airways

Beginning of inspiration

Intrathoracic airway

Alveolus 0

0   0

Intrapleural space −0.5

During forced expiration

8.7   8 6   4   0

+8.0

Numbers are pressures in kPa (1 kPa = 7.5 mmHg)

(c) The effect of effort on inspiratory and expiratory airflow

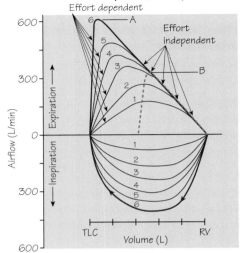

Effort dependent

Effort independent

Airflow (L/min)
Expiration
Inspiration

A
B

TLC   Volume (L)   RV

- - - - = Flow–volume curve for maximum effort from partly filled lungs
A = Peak expiratory flow rate with lungs filled to total lung capacity
B = Peak expiratory flow rate for partly filled lungs filled (RV + 3 L)
TLC = Total lung capacity, RV = Residual volume

(e) Maximum flow–volume loops

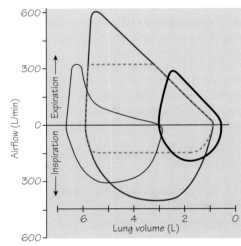

Airflow (L/min)
Expiration
Inspiration

6   4   2   0
Lung volume (L)

— **Normal curve**

— **Obstructive airway disease of smaller airways.** Note:
  • concave appearance of forced expiratory curve
  • forced inspiratory flow affected less than forced expiratory flow

- - - **Upper airway obstruction (e.g. tracheal stenosis).** Note:
  • flat topped flow–volume curve
  • forced inspiratory flow affected as much as expiratory flow

— **Restrictive lung disease.** Low peak flow rates are related to low volume. (Note: this figure is drawn to show the relationship between these traces by using absolute lung volume which cannot actually be obtained from a flow–volume loop alone).

Airflow is driven by the mouth–alveolar pressure gradient generated by the respiratory muscles (Chapters 2 and 3).

$$\text{Airflow} = \frac{\Delta P(= \text{mouth} - \text{alveolar pressure})}{\text{RAW}(= \text{resistance of the airways})}$$

In **laminar flow**, gas particles move parallel to the walls, with centre layers moving faster than outer ones, creating a cone-shaped front (Fig. 7a). The factors affecting laminar flow of a fluid of viscosity, η, in smooth straight tubes of length, l, and radius, r, are described in **Poiseuille's equation**:

$$\text{Flow} = \frac{\Delta P}{R} = \Delta P \frac{\pi r^4}{8\ell\eta} \quad \therefore R = \frac{8\ell\eta}{\pi r^4}$$

Halving the radius of an airway increases its resistance 16-fold. However, although the resistance of an individual bronchiole is high, there are thousands in parallel. The total resistance of each generation of peripheral airways is normally low, and the overall resistance of lung airways is dominated by the larger airways. Outside the lung, the nose and pharynx contribute substantial resistance, which can be reduced by mouth breathing, for example, during exercise. Peripheral airways are often affected by disease, but because their resistance must increase considerably to measurably affect airway resistance (RAW), they are known as the **silent zone**.

At higher linear velocities, especially in wide airways and near branch points, flow may become **turbulent**. With turbulence, the wave front is square and flow $\propto \sqrt{\Delta P}$ (not ΔP), reflecting the dissipation of energy in the formation of eddies. Normally, at rest, flow is laminar throughout the airways, but in exercise it may become turbulent, especially in the trachea, generating characteristic harsh breath sounds.

Factors affecting airway resistance
Bronchial smooth muscle and epithelium

Bronchial smooth muscle (Fig. 7b) receives a **parasympathetic bronchoconstrictor** nerve supply, acting via acetylcholine and muscarinic type 3 receptors, which forms the efferent limb of a reflex from airway irritant receptors (rapidly adapting receptors). The smooth muscle also contains β_2-adrenergic receptors, which cause relaxation when stimulated by circulating **epinephrine** (adrenaline) or drugs such as salbutamol. Sympathetic innervation of the airways is sparse in humans and has little effect on airway smooth muscle. Airways are also supplied with excitatory and inhibitory non-adrenergic non-cholinergic (NANC) nerves, the former acting via the transmitters substance P and neurokinins, and the latter via nitric oxide (NO) and/or VIP (vasoactive intestinal peptide). Parasympathetic bronchoconstriction is inhibited by activation of airway stretch receptors (slowly adapting receptors), and CO_2 has a direct bronchodilator effect. Pollutants (e.g. sulphur dioxide and ozone) and substances released from mast cells and eosinophils can increase RAW via bronchoconstriction, mucosal oedema, mucus hypersecretion, mucus plugging and epithelial shedding – all of which are important in asthma (Chapter 24). Airway resistance can also be increased by chronic mucosal hypertrophy in chronic obstructive pulmonary disease (COPD) (Chapter 26) and by material within the airways, such as inhaled foreign bodies or tumours (Chapter 40).

Transmural (airway–intrapleural) pressure gradient
The pressure difference across airways can have important effects on their calibre, and this underlies the effects of effort on airflow,

illustrated in Fig. 7c. Airflow is measured continuously and plotted against lung volume as the subject breathes between residual volume (RV) and total lung capacity (TLC). The inspiratory airflow at any volume increases progressively with increasing effort (1 = minimum effort, 6 = maximum effort). The flow–volume curves for progressively increasing expiratory efforts (upper traces 1–6) are more complicated. In the early part of expiration from TLC, flow is **effort-dependent**, but towards the end of the breath, as volume declines, the traces produced at different effort levels come together. Expiratory airflow towards the end of a breath is **effort-independent** and determined by lung volume. **Peak expiratory flow rate** (PEFR) is seen to be reduced (B in Fig. 7c) if the lungs are only partially filled at the start of the forced expiration.

Effort-independent airflow is explained by **dynamic compression of airways**. Before the start of inspiration (Fig. 7d, upper panel) the pressure along the airways is zero, intrapleural pressure is negative (Chapter 3) and transmural pressure acts to hold airways open. Intrapleural pressure is negative during both quiet and forced inspiration and it remains negative in quiet expiration, so transmural pressure holds airways open. In a forced expiration, however, expiratory muscle contraction raises intrapleural pressure well above atmospheric pressure (e.g. 8 kPa, 60 mmHg), increasing the pressure gradient from alveoli to mouth. This would be expected to increase airflow, but the increased intrapleural pressure also acts to compress airways. Airway pressure falls progressively along the airway, and at some point – usually in the bronchi – the airway pressure will be sufficiently below intrapleural pressure for the airway to collapse, despite its cartilaginous support. Pressure will then build up distally, opening the airways again. The resulting fluttering walls can be seen on bronchoscopy and produce the brassy note audible on forced expiration in healthy people.

RAW in disease
Increased airway resistance is important in many diseases and can be measured using a body plethysmograph. In healthy individuals, RAW is about 0.2 kPa/L per second (1.5 mmHg/L per second). More commonly, airway resistance is assessed indirectly from forced expiratory measurements, such as **forced expiratory volume in 1 second** (FEV$_1$), **forced vital capacity** (FVC) and PEFR (Chapter 20). Especially useful is the **forced expiratory ratio** (FER = FEV$_1$/FVC), which is reduced when RAW is increased in **obstructive pulmonary disease**. High airway resistance accentuates dynamic compression of airways by augmenting the pressure drop along airways. In addition, the airways may be less able to resist compression, in emphysema because of reduced radial traction and in asthma because of bronchoconstriction. Collapse of small airways may occur, leading to incomplete expiration, **air trapping** and increased functional residual capacity. Inability to produce high expiratory airflow impairs effective coughing, which can lead to a vicious cycle as secretions accumulate, further increasing RAW and further reducing peak flow. **Expiratory wheezes (rhonchi)**, heard in asthma and other obstructive diseases, are probably generated by oscillations in opposing airway walls near their point of closure, like sounds from the reeds of an oboe. A reasonable airflow is needed to generate such sounds, and when constriction becomes very severe, they disappear to give the ominous silent chest seen in life-threatening asthma. Small airway collapse leads to characteristic shape of the maximum flow–volume curve in obstructive airway disease (Fig. 7e), which differs from that in upper airway obstruction and restrictive lung disease.

8 Carriage of oxygen

(a) Haemoglobin structure

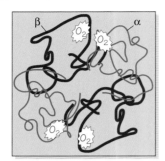

Haemoglobin is composed of four subunits, each containing a protein chain (globin) and a haem group. Normal adult haemoglobin, HbA, contains two identical α-chains composed of 141 amino acids and two β-chains composed of 146 amino acids. The haem group ( ) is attached to each chain at a histidine residue, and each has an iron atom in the ferrous form, which binds to an oxygen molecule. The haem groups lie in crevices in the crumpled ball of globin chains. The exact 3D (or quaternary) structure of haemoglobin can change and alter the accessibility of the oxygen-binding site. Each molecule of haemoglobin can bind up to four molecules of oxygen in a series of reactions which can be summarized as:

$$Hb_4 + 4O_2 \Leftrightarrow Hb_4(O_2)_4$$

(b) The oxygen–haemoglobin dissociation curve, haemoglobin concentration (150 g/L)

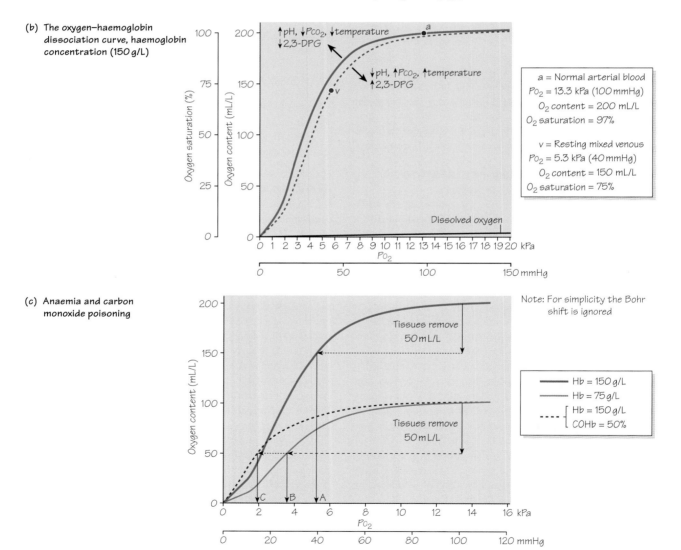

↑pH, ↓P_{CO_2}, ↓temperature ↓2,3-DPG

↓pH, ↑P_{CO_2}, ↑temperature ↑2,3-DPG

a = Normal arterial blood
P_{O_2} = 13.3 kPa (100 mmHg)
O_2 content = 200 mL/L
O_2 saturation = 97%

v = Resting mixed venous
P_{O_2} = 5.3 kPa (40 mmHg)
O_2 content = 150 mL/L
O_2 saturation = 75%

Dissolved oxygen

(c) Anaemia and carbon monoxide poisoning

Note: For simplicity the Bohr shift is ignored

Tissues remove 50 mL/L

Tissues remove 50 mL/L

Hb = 150 g/L
Hb = 75 g/L
Hb = 150 g/L
COHb = 50%

At rest, a man consumes about 250 mL oxygen/min, which may rise to more than 4000 mL/min in exercise if he is very fit. Oxygen diffuses from alveolus to blood until equilibrium is reached when pulmonary capillary P_{O_2} equals alveolar P_{O_2}. The **solubility** of oxygen in blood is low – 0.000225 mL oxygen per mL of blood per kPa (0.00003 mL/mL/mmHg) – so that at a normal arterial P_{O_2} of 13.3 kPa (100 mmHg) there is only 3 mL dissolved in each litre of blood. The main function of the red blood cell pigment, **haemoglobin**, the key features of whose structure is shown in Fig. 8a, is to carry the large quantities of oxygen needed by the tissues.

Each gram of haemoglobin combines with up to 1.34 mL oxygen, so with a haemoglobin concentration, [Hb], of 150 g/L, blood contains a maximum of 200 mL/L oxygen bound to haemoglobin. This is known as the **oxygen capacity**, which varies with [Hb]. The actual amount of oxygen bound also depends on the P_{O_2}. The percentage of the available binding sites bound to oxygen is known as the **oxygen saturation**.

Oxygen saturation:

$$\frac{\text{Amount of oxygen bound to haemoglobin (mL/L)}}{\text{Oxygen capacity (mL/L)}} \times 100\%$$

The oxygen content of the blood (mL/L) equals the sum of haemoglobin-bound oxygen and the small amount of dissolved oxygen. The rate of rise of oxygen content with increasing partial pressure depends on the number of free haemoglobin-binding sites remaining and their affinity for oxygen. As each oxygen molecule binds in turn to the four haem groups, the quaternary structure alters and the affinity of the remaining binding sites for oxygen increases. This **cooperative binding** increases the steepness of the **oxygen–haemoglobin dissociation curve** in the middle (Fig. 8b), but the curve flattens again at partial pressures above about 8 kPa (60 mmHg) because there are few unfilled binding sites remaining. In arterial blood, P_{O_2} is normally about 13 kPa (100 mmHg), oxygen saturation about 97%, and, with a normal [Hb], an oxygen content of about 200 mL/L. Rises or modest falls in P_{O_2} from 13 kPa (100 mmHg), for example during hyperventilation or mild hypoventilation, cause little change in the arterial oxygen content, as the dissociation curve is flat in this region. More severe reductions in P_{O_2}, to levels in the steep region (<8 kPa, 60 mmHg), are associated with significant reductions in oxygen saturation and content. Consequently, breathing oxygen-enriched air may significantly raise arterial oxygen content and hence exercise capacity at high altitude and in patients with chronic hypoxic respiratory disease, but has little effect on a healthy person at sea level.

Low P_{O_2} in tissue capillaries causes oxygen release from haemoglobin, whereas the high P_{O_2} in pulmonary capillaries causes oxygen binding. The affinity of haemoglobin for oxygen, and hence the position of the dissociation curve, varies with local conditions. A reduced oxygen affinity, shown by a right shift in the curve, is caused by a fall in pH, a rise in P_{CO_2} (the **Bohr effect**) or increased temperature (Fig. 8b). These changes occur in metabolically active tissues such as exercising muscle and encourage oxygen release. In the lungs, oxygen uptake is aided by the increasing affinity of haemoglobin for oxygen, caused by falling P_{CO_2} and temperature and increased pH and reflected by a left shift of the curve. The P_{O_2} at which the haemoglobin is 50% saturated is known as the P_{50}. Under normal arterial conditions (pH = 7.4, P_{CO_2} = 5.3 kPa or 40 mmHg, temperature = 37°C) P_{50} = 3.5 kPa (26.3 mmHg); right shifts raise the P_{50} and left shifts lower it. A rise in the concentration of **2,3-di(or bi)phosphoglycerate** (2,3-DPG), which is a by-product of glycolysis in red cells, also causes a right shift. A rise in 2,3-DPG occurs in anaemia, causing a modest increase in P_{50}. Blood bank storage causes progressive depletion of 2,3-DPG and an undesirable left shift, but this can be minimized by storing the blood with citrate-phosphate-dextrose.

Anaemia and carbon monoxide poisoning

In **anaemia**, at any given P_{O_2}, the oxygen content is reduced because of the reduced concentration of binding sites. Figure 8c shows the dissociation curve for normal blood and for blood with [Hb] = 75g/L. Alveolar and arterial P_{O_2} is normal in anaemia and therefore arterial O_2 content is 100 mL/L. At rest, the tissues need to remove about 50 mL/L of oxygen from the blood passing through them. To achieve this mixed venous content, P_{O_2} will need to fall to about 5.3 kPa (40 mmHg) (A in Fig. 8c) when [Hb] = 150 g/L and about 3.6 kPa (27 mmHg) (B) when [Hb] = 75 g/L. The reduced venous and hence capillary P_{O_2} reduces the partial pressure gradient driving diffusion of oxygen to the tissues, which is adequate at rest but which may become inadequate in exercise when oxygen consumption increases.

Figure 8c also shows the dissociation curve for blood that has 50% of oxygen-binding sites occupied by carbon monoxide (CO, dashed line). Arterial oxygen content is 100 mL/L, but there is also an altered shape and leftward shift of the dissociation curve, because CO binding increases the affinity of the remaining (CO-free) sites for oxygen. This impairs oxygen release in the tissues. Mixed venous P_{O_2} will now have to fall to 2 kPa (15 mmHg) (point C) to release the 50 mL/L required, and this will greatly reduce the pressure gradient for diffusion. At about 50–60% **carboxyhaemoglobin**, symptoms of impaired cerebral oxygenation (headache, convulsions, coma and death) are severe, whereas anaemic patients with the same arterial oxygen content are typically asymptomatic at rest. Haemoglobin has a high affinity for CO (~240 times that for oxygen), so breathing even at low concentrations causes a progressive increase in the cherry-red carboxyhaemoglobin. A cherry-red complexion is sometimes a feature of CO poisoning, although pallor and **cyanosis** (discussed in Chapter 23) are more common.

Other respiratory pigments

Fetal haemoglobin, HbF, differs from **adult haemoglobin, HbA**, in that there are two γ-chains instead of two β-chains. The HbF dissociation curve lies to the left of that for HbA, reflecting its higher O_2 affinity. This difference is enhanced by the **double Bohr shift**: in the placenta P_{CO_2} moves from the fetal to maternal blood, shifting the maternal curve further right and the fetal curve further left. The high affinity of HbF relative to HbA helps transfer oxygen from mother to fetus, and even though blood returning from the placenta to the fetus in the umbilical vein has a P_{O_2} of only about 4 kPa (30 mmHg), its saturation is 70%. Oxygen transport in the fetus is also helped by a high [Hb] of about 170–180 g/L.

Myoglobin, the respiratory pigment found in muscle, is composed of a single haem group attached to a single globin chain. With no cooperative binding, its dissociation curve is hyperbolic. It is also far to the left of HbA and its high affinity means that its oxygen store is only released when local P_{O_2} is severely reduced, for example in heavy exercise.

⑨ Carriage of carbon dioxide

(a) CO_2 dissociation curve

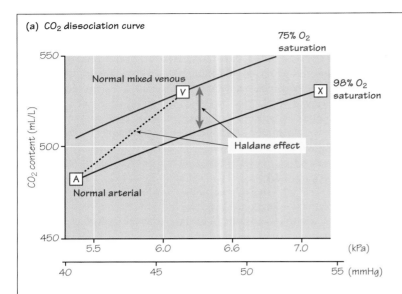

The red line (**A-X**) shows what the relationship between blood PCO_2 and CO_2 content would be if Hb remained 98% saturated. However, as mixed venous blood HB is only 75% saturated, more CO_2 can be carried for any given PCO_2, as shown by the dashed line **A-V** (the Haldane effect, see box and text).

(c) How CO_2 is carried in arterial and venous blood

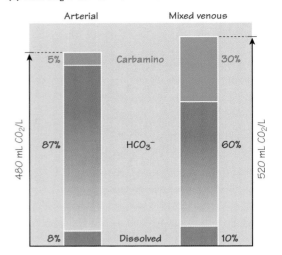

(b) CO_2 uptake and O_2 delivery in the tissues — role of red cells

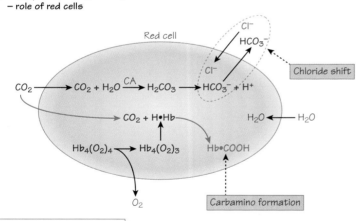

CA = carbonic anhydrase
Hb = haemoglobin subunit
H•Hb = reduced haemoglobin

The basis of the Haldane effect

When haemoglobin is fully oxygenated, each of the four Hb subunits is bound to one O_2: $Hb_4(O_2)_4$
As O_2 is released, i.e.

$$Hb_4(O_2)_4 \longrightarrow Hb_4(O_2)_3 \longrightarrow Hb_4(O_2)_2 \longrightarrow Hb_4(O_2)$$

the ability of each reduced (deoxygenated) Hb subunit (H•Hb) to buffer H^+ and form Hb•COOH (carbaminohaemoglobin) is greatly increased

This enhances carriage of CO_2 by blood by:
(a) buffering red cell acidity and therefore facilitating formation of HCO_3^-
(b) formation of Hb•COOH

When blood is reoxygenated in the lungs, the reverse occurs, facilitating removal of CO_2 in the breath

 The Respiratory System at a Glance, 3e. By J.P.T. Ward, J. Ward, R.M. Leach. Published 2010 Blackwell Publishing Ltd.

Carbon dioxide (CO_2) is produced by tissues and transported in the blood to the lungs, where it is expired. The amount of CO_2 that can be carried in the blood is much greater than that of O_2, as seen in the **CO_2 dissociation curve** (Fig. 9a). The CO_2 dissociation curve is also more linear and does not reach a plateau. CO_2 is transported in the blood as bicarbonate ions, as carbamino compounds combined with proteins or simply dissolved in the plasma (Fig. 9b).

Bicarbonate: In mixed venous blood about 60% of CO_2 is transported in the form of bicarbonate. CO_2 and water combine to form carbonic acid (H_2CO_3) and thence bicarbonate (HCO_3^-):

$$CO_2 + H_2O \overset{CA}{\Leftrightarrow} H_2CO_3 \Leftrightarrow H^+ + HCO_3^- \qquad (1)$$

The left-hand side of the equation proceeds slowly in plasma, but is accelerated dramatically by the enzyme **carbonic anhydrase** (CA), which is present in red blood cells. Ionization of carbonic acid to bicarbonate and H^+ is rapid in the absence of any enzyme. Bicarbonate is therefore formed preferentially in the red cells, from which it easily diffuses out into the plasma. The red cell membrane is however impermeable to H^+ ions and they remain within the cell. To maintain electrical neutrality, Cl^- ions diffuse into the cell to replace bicarbonate, an effect known as the **chloride shift** (Fig. 9c). A build-up of H^+ in the red blood cell would impair further movement of Equation 1 to the right, thus limiting formation of bicarbonate. However, H^+ binds avidly to reduced (deoxygenated) haemoglobin; i.e. **haemoglobin acts as a buffer**, so the rise in H^+ concentration is limited and more bicarbonate can be formed. Oxygenated haemoglobin does not bind H^+ so well, as it is more acidic. This contributes to the **Haldane effect**, which states that, for any given P_{CO_2}, the CO_2 content of deoxygenated blood is greater than that of oxygenated blood. As a result, when blood gives up oxygen to respiring tissues, i.e. becomes deoxygenated, it is able to take up more of the CO_2 that the tissues are producing. Conversely, oxygenation of haemoglobin in the lung assists the unloading of CO_2 from the blood so it can be expired. This is illustrated in Fig. 9a and Equation 2.

$$H^+ + haemoglobin \cdot O_2 \Leftrightarrow haemoglobin \cdot H + O_2 \qquad (2)$$

Note that as a consequence of all the above, deoxygenated red blood cells have a higher intracellular osmolality and water enters, causing them to swell slightly. In the lung, CO_2 is given off, osmolality falls and the red cells shrink again.

Carbamino compounds: CO_2 combines rapidly with terminal amino groups on proteins to form carbamino compounds:

$$CO_2 + protein \cdot NH_2 \Leftrightarrow protein \cdot NH \cdot COOH \qquad (3)$$

In blood, the most prevalent protein is haemoglobin, which combines with CO_2 to form carbaminohaemoglobin. Reduced haemoglobin forms carbamino compounds more readily than oxygenated haemoglobin, and this also contributes to the Haldane effect (Fig. 9b). About 30% of the CO_2 expired is carried to the lungs as carbamino compounds.

CO_2 in solution: CO_2 is approximately 20 times more soluble in water than O_2. A significant proportion ($\sim$10%) of the CO_2 exhaled is therefore carried to the lung dissolved in the plasma.

Because of the Haldane effect, the proportion of CO_2 that is carried in the blood as bicarbonate, carbamino compounds and simply dissolved differs between oxygenated arterial blood and deoxygenated mixed venous blood (Fig. 9b).

Hypoventilation and hyperventilation

Ventilation is normally closely matched to the metabolic requirements of the body, and this can be estimated from the rate of CO_2 production (Chapter 11). The partial pressure of CO_2 in the alveoli ($P_{A}CO_2$) is proportional to the amount of CO_2 exhaled per minute (V_{CO_2}) as a fraction of total alveolar ventilation (V_A), i.e. $P_{A}CO_2 \propto V_{CO_2}/V_A$. The gas in the alveoli is in equilibrium with arterial blood, so $P_{A}CO_2$ estimates the partial pressure in the blood ($P_{a}CO_2$). At any given metabolic rate, doubling the alveolar ventilation halves alveolar and arterial P_{CO_2}, and halving alveolar ventilation doubles $P_{A}CO_2$ and $P_{a}CO_2$. Changes in alveolar ventilation also affect alveolar P_{O_2}, but the relationship is not as simple because O_2 is present in both inspired and expired gas. Thus, doubling alveolar ventilation will halve the *difference* between the inspired and alveolar O_2 fraction. **Hypoventilation** (underventilation) and **hyperventilation** (overventilation) are therefore defined in terms of $P_{a}CO_2$, so that a patient is *hypoventilating* when $P_{a}CO_2$ is more than 45 mmHg (5.9 kPa) and *hyperventilating* when the $P_{a}CO_2$ is less than 40 mmHg (5.3 kPa). Note that the CO_2 content of the blood will be affected more slowly by hypo- or hyperventilation than the O_2 content, as the CO_2 stores in the body (e.g. as HCO_3^-) are approximately 75 times greater than those for O_2 (e.g. haemoglobin and myoglobin). Also, although hyperventilation increases arterial P_{O_2}, in a healthy patient it has little effect on O_2 content as arterial haemoglobin is normally close to saturation (Chapter 8).

Hypoventilation may occur when the respiratory drive is impaired by head injury, or drugs such as morphine or barbiturates which suppress the respiratory centres. It may also be caused by respiratory muscle weakness or severe chest trauma. Hypoventilation is sometimes a feature of severe chronic obstructive airways disease (COPD; Chapter 26), but is not usually a feature of asthma (Chapter 25) unless the attack is severe or prolonged enough to lead to exhaustion. Hypoventilation is difficult to achieve voluntarily, as the respiratory centres create an overwhelming desire to breathe.

Hypoventilation leads to **hypercapnia** (high $P_{a}CO_2$) and **hypoxia** (low $P_{a}O_2$). Increasing severity of hypercapnia causes peripheral vasodilatation, muscle twitching and hand flap, confusion, drowsiness and eventually coma; there is a concomitant respiratory acidosis (Chapter 10). The effects of hypoxia are dealt with elsewhere (Chapter 8). Hyperventilation can be induced voluntarily and in states of high anxiety (e.g. panic attacks) or pain. It results in a low $P_{a}CO_2$ (**hypocapnia**), which can cause light-headedness, visual disturbances due to cerebral vasoconstriction, paraesthesia ('pins and needles') and muscle cramps, especially carpopedal spasm; there is a concomitant respiratory alkalosis (Chapter 10).

Respiratory gas exchange ratio

Respiratory gas exchange ratio (R) is the ratio of CO_2 production to O_2 consumption as measured at the mouth. In the steady state, CO_2 production and O_2 consumption reflect tissue metabolism. Metabolizing carbohydrates produces a volume of CO_2 equal to the volume of O_2 consumed, whereas metabolizing fats and proteins produces a smaller volume of CO_2 than O_2 consumed. For an average mixed diet R $\approx$ 0.8.

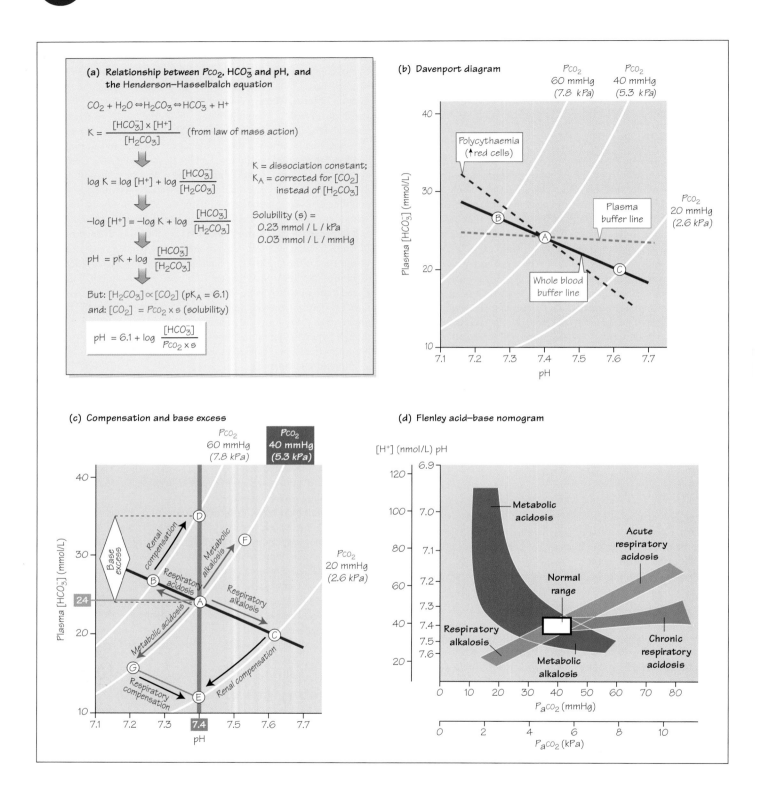

(a) Relationship between P_{CO_2}, HCO_3^- and pH, and the Henderson–Hasselbalch equation

$$CO_2 + H_2O \rightleftharpoons H_2CO_3 \rightleftharpoons HCO_3^- + H^+$$

$$K = \frac{[HCO_3^-] \times [H^+]}{[H_2CO_3]} \quad \text{(from law of mass action)}$$

$$\log K = \log [H^+] + \log \frac{[HCO_3^-]}{[H_2CO_3]}$$

$$-\log [H^+] = -\log K + \log \frac{[HCO_3^-]}{[H_2CO_3]}$$

$$pH = pK + \log \frac{[HCO_3^-]}{[H_2CO_3]}$$

But: $[H_2CO_3] \propto [CO_2]$ ($pK_A = 6.1$)
and: $[CO_2] = P_{CO_2} \times s$ (solubility)

$$pH = 6.1 + \log \frac{[HCO_3^-]}{P_{CO_2} \times s}$$

K = dissociation constant;
K_A = corrected for $[CO_2]$ instead of $[H_2CO_3]$

Solubility (s) =
0.23 mmol / L / kPa
0.03 mmol / L / mmHg

(b) Davenport diagram

(c) Compensation and base excess

(d) Flenley acid–base nomogram

The pH of arterial blood is normally approximately 7.4 ($[H^+] = 40$ nmol/L). Regulation of **acid–base status** so that blood pH remains between 7.35 and 7.45 (45–35 nmol/L) is vital for the correct functioning of the body. Carriage of CO_2 in blood and its removal in the lungs (Chapter 9) have an important influence on acid–base status, as about 100 times more acid equivalents are expired per day in the form of CO_2/carbonic acid than are excreted as fixed acids by the kidneys. Nevertheless, renal mechanisms are crucially important for regulation of acid–base balance, and for compensating respiratory disorders (see below).

Buffers bind or release H^+ according to the pH; this limits the change in pH that occurs when acid is added. The relationship between the amount of acid equivalent added to a solution containing a buffer and the resultant change in pH is known as the **buffer curve**. Buffers are most effective when pH is close to their pK_A (log of dissociation constant, K_A; see Fig. 10a). The most important buffers in blood are **bicarbonate** (HCO_3^-) and **haemoglobin**. CO_2 combines with water to form carbonic acid (H_2CO_3), which dissociates to HCO_3^- and H^+ (Chapter 9). The relationship between pH, P_{CO_2} and $[HCO_3^-]$ is described by the **Henderson–Hasselbalch equation** (Fig. 10a), where pK_A is 6.1 and $[CO_2]$ can be calculated as $P_{CO_2} \times CO_2$ solubility, which is 0.03 mmol L/mmHg (0.23 mmol L/kPa). In normal blood, $[HCO_3^-]$ is 24 mmol and P_{CO_2} 40 mmHg (5.3 kPa), and pH calculates as 7.4. Whatever their actual values, the important points to remember are that if the ratio $[HCO_3^-]/[CO_2]$ remains constant at 20, then pH will remain at 7.4, and:

$$pH \propto \log \frac{[HCO_3^-]}{P_{CO_2}}$$

Although the pK_A of the bicarbonate system (6.1) is further away from blood pH (7.4) than would seem ideal for a buffer, the fact that P_{CO_2} and HCO_3^- can be independently controlled by ventilation (Chapter 9) and the kidneys, respectively, means that in practice it makes an effective buffer system.

Haemoglobin is an important buffer, particularly when deoxygenated (Chapter 9), and significantly improves the buffering capacity of whole blood compared with plasma (Fig. 10b; the steeper the line, the better the buffering). All other **blood proteins** combined have slightly more than 20% of the buffering capacity of haemoglobin.

Acidosis, alkalosis and compensation

The relationship between pH, HCO_3^- and P_{CO_2} can be portrayed using a **Davenport diagram** (Fig. 10b). HCO_3^- is plotted against pH for given values of P_{CO_2}. The line marked BAC is the **buffer line** for whole blood; in the absence of other changes (e.g. anaemia and polycythaemia), changes in P_{CO_2} alter HCO_3^- and pH along this line. Point A represents normal conditions (pH 7.4, HCO_3^- 24 mmol, P_{CO_2} 40 mmHg/5.3 kPa). An acute rise in P_{CO_2} (hypercapnia) due to hypoventilation (e.g. **acute respiratory failure**) will decrease the $[HCO_3^-]$: P_{CO_2} ratio and consequently pH (see above). This **respiratory acidosis** is represented by a move from A to B (Fig. 10c); points A to C represent a **respiratory alkalosis** (e.g. hyperventilation). A sustained respiratory acidosis caused by **chronic respiratory failure** (Chapter 23) can over days be partially **compensated** by excretion of H^+ (as phosphate and ammonium) and reabsorption of HCO_3^- in the kidneys. The $[HCO_3^-]/P_{CO_2}$ ratio is thus largely restored and pH returns

towards normal. This **renal compensation** is described by the arrow between B and D (Fig. 10c). Conversely, a respiratory alkalosis may be compensated by increased renal excretion of HCO_3^- (C to E).

The term **metabolic acidosis** (or **alkalosis**) is used when acid–base status is disturbed by changes in HCO_3^- rather than CO_2 – as a result, for example, of renal disease or increased H^+ production (table). A **metabolic acidosis** (Fig. 10c, G) may be partially compensated by increased ventilation and a reduction in P_{CO_2} (G to E), initiated by detection of acid pH by the chemoreceptors (Chapter 11). There can be little **respiratory compensation** for **metabolic alkalosis** (F), as this may require unsustainable falls in ventilation.

Base excess

Measurement of pH alone therefore gives little indication of acid–base status (Fig. 10d); although pH may be normal, P_{CO_2} and $[HCO_3^-]$ may not be (D, E). Measurements of blood pH, P_{CO_2} and P_{O_2} are always taken clinically. **Base excess** (or **base deficit** – negative base excess) is a *calculated* value representing the amount of acid that would be needed to titrate the blood back to a pH of 7.4 at a P_{CO_2} of 5.3 kPa. For example, in Fig. 10c an increase in P_{CO_2} to 60 mmHg results in a respiratory acidosis (B). Full compensation back to pH 7.4 (D) requires $[HCO_3^-]$ to be increased to approximately 35 mmol/L; thus following renal compensation (D), the base excess is approximately 11 mmol/L (the difference between A and D). In a pure metabolic acidosis, the base excess is negative and greater than the difference between the actual and normal HCO_3^-, as haemoglobin and buffers must also be titrated. Base excess is normally calculated from the pH and P_{CO_2} automatically by clinical blood gas analysers, and corrected for haemoglobin concentration. Together with the P_{CO_2}, base excess may be useful for diagnosis of the cause of an acid–base disturbance, but should be used with caution as a basis for treatment as the whole-body buffer line may differ significantly from that of blood *in vitro*, due to contributions from interstitial fluids (Fig. 10b).

Metabolic and respiratory acid–base disorders may often be combined, making diagnosis difficult. A common example is respiratory failure (Chapter 23), where concomitant hypoxia can cause metabolic acidosis in addition to the primary respiratory acidosis. A useful diagnostic aid is the **Flenley nomogram** (Fig. 10d). Only one type of disturbance is likely if the patient's arterial pH and P_{CO_2} fall within a band (95% confidence limits).

Common causes of acid–base disorders

Respiratory acidosis	Respiratory alkalosis
Airway obstruction	High levels of anxiety
Respiratory muscle disease	(hyperventilation)
Head trauma	Pain
	Altitude
	Excessive mechanical ventilation
Metabolic acidosis	**Metabolic alkalosis**
Loss of HCO_3^- from gut (diarrhoea)	Volume depletion
Renal failure or tubular damage	Diuretics (loop, thiazide)
Lactic acidosis (hypoxia, sepsis)	K^+ deficiency
Ketoacidosis (diabetes, starvation)	Excess mineralocorticoids
	Vomiting, loss of stomach fluids

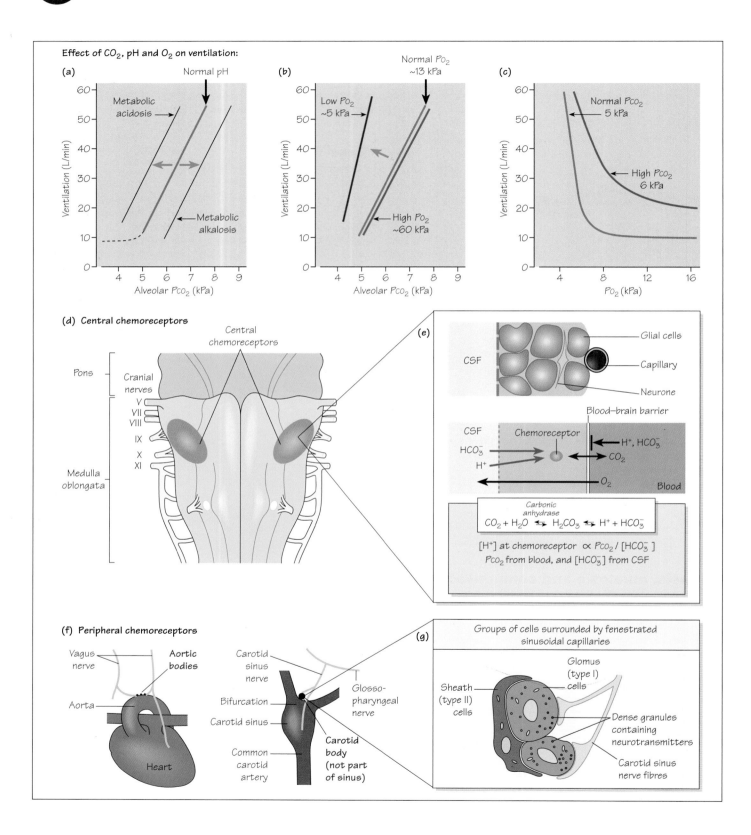

Effect of CO_2, pH and O_2 on ventilation:

(a) Metabolic acidosis / Normal pH / Metabolic alkalosis — Ventilation (L/min) vs Alveolar P_{CO_2} (kPa)

(b) Low P_{O_2} ~5 kPa / Normal P_{O_2} ~13 kPa / High P_{O_2} ~60 kPa — Ventilation (L/min) vs Alveolar P_{CO_2} (kPa)

(c) Normal P_{CO_2} 5 kPa / High P_{CO_2} 6 kPa — Ventilation (L/min) vs P_{O_2} (kPa)

(d) Central chemoreceptors

(e) Glial cells / Capillary / Neurone / CSF

Blood–brain barrier / CSF / Chemoreceptor / HCO_3^- / H^+ / H^+, HCO_3^- / CO_2 / O_2 / Blood

Carbonic anhydrase
$$CO_2 + H_2O \leftrightarrows H_2CO_3 \leftrightarrows H^+ + HCO_3^-$$

$[H^+]$ at chemoreceptor $\propto P_{CO_2} / [HCO_3^-]$
P_{CO_2} from blood, and $[HCO_3^-]$ from CSF

(f) Peripheral chemoreceptors

(g) Groups of cells surrounded by fenestrated sinusoidal capillaries

Chemical control of ventilation is mediated via **central** and **peripheral chemoreceptors**, which detect arterial P_{CO_2} and pH (central and peripheral) and P_{O_2} (peripheral only), and modulate ventilation via a distributed network of neurones in the **brainstem** (Chapter 12). P_{CO_2} is the most important factor. The chemoreceptors allow arterial P_{CO_2} and P_{O_2} to be maintained within narrow limits despite large changes in metabolism (e.g. exercise), although ventilation in exercise is also affected by other factors (Chapter 15).

Ventilatory response to changes in $P_{A_{CO_2}}$ and $P_{A_{O_2}}$

Normal alveolar P_{CO_2} ($P_{A_{CO_2}}$) is approximately 5.3 kPa (40 mmHg). Increasing $P_{A_{CO_2}}$ causes minute ventilation (litres ventilated per minute) to rise in an almost linear fashion (Fig. 11a), by approximately 15–25 L/min for each kPa rise in $P_{A_{CO_2}}$ ($\sim$2.7 L/min per mmHg). There is considerable variation between individuals, and athletes and patients with chronic respiratory disease often have a reduced response to $P_{A_{CO_2}}$ (Chapters 26 and 44). If $P_{A_{CO_2}}$ increases above 10 kPa, ventilation decreases due to direct suppression of central respiratory neurones. A **metabolic acidosis** (an increase in [H^+] caused by reduced [HCO_3^-]; see Chapter 10) shifts the CO_2–ventilation response curve to the left, whereas a **metabolic alkalosis** shifts it to the right (Fig. 11a). Note that a rise in [H^+] caused by increased P_{CO_2} is called a **respiratory acidosis**. Increasing $P_{A_{O_2}}$ from the normal value of approximately 13 kPa ($\sim$100 mmHg) has little effect on the CO_2–ventilation response curve, but if the $P_{A_{O_2}}$ is reduced, the slope of the relationship becomes steeper and ventilation increases more for any given rise in $P_{A_{CO_2}}$ (Fig. 11b). When the effect of $P_{A_{CO_2}}$ is investigated independently (at constant $P_{A_{CO_2}}$), there is little increase in ventilation until the $P_{A_{O_2}}$ falls below approximately 8 kPa ($\sim$60 mmHg) (Fig. 11c). The effect of reducing $P_{A_{O_2}}$ is however potentiated if the $P_{A_{CO_2}}$ is raised – i.e. there is a **synergistic** (more than additive) relationship between the effects of $P_{A_{O_2}}$ and $P_{A_{CO_2}}$.

The central chemoreceptor

The **central chemoreceptor** consists of a diffuse collection of neurones located near the ventrolateral surface of the medulla, close to the exit of IX and X cranial nerves (Fig. 11d). These are sensitive to the pH of the surrounding cerebrospinal fluid (CSF) and do **not** respond to P_{O_2}. CSF is separated from blood by the **blood–brain barrier**, a tight endothelial layer lining the blood vessels of the brain. This barrier is impermeable to polar (charged) molecules such as H^+ and HCO_3^-, but CO_2 can diffuse across it easily. The pH of CSF is therefore determined by the arterial P_{CO_2} and the CSF [HCO_3^-] (Chapter 10), and is not directly affected by changes in blood pH (Fig. 11e). CSF contains little protein, so its buffering capacity is low; therefore, a small change in P_{CO_2} will cause a large change in pH. Stimulation of the central chemoreceptor by a fall in CSF pH (rise in blood P_{CO_2}) causes an increase in ventilation. The central chemoreceptor is thought to be responsible for approximately 80% of the response to CO_2 in humans.

It has a relatively slow response time ($\sim$20 seconds), as CO_2 has to diffuse across the blood–brain barrier.

The peripheral chemoreceptors

The **peripheral chemoreceptors** are within the **carotid** and **aortic bodies**. The carotid body is a small ($\sim$2 mg) structure located at the bifurcation of the common carotid artery, just above the carotid sinus. It is innervated by the carotid sinus nerve, leading to the glossopharyngeal (Fig. 11f). The aortic bodies are distributed around the aortic arch and are innervated by the vagus. In humans, they are much less important than carotid bodies. The carotid body contains **glomus** (type I) cells and **sheath** (type II) cells (Fig. 11g). Glomus cells are responsible for chemoreception; they have dense granules containing neurotransmitters and contact axons of the carotid sinus nerve. The function of sheath cells may be to protect and support the glomus cells, analogous to glial cells in the central nervous system.

Carotid bodies respond to increased P_{CO_2} or [H^+] and decreased P_{O_2} (**not** blood O_2 content) by increasing firing rate in the carotid sinus nerve, and thus ventilation. They have a high blood flow and consequently a small arteriovenous difference for P_{CO_2} and P_{O_2}. They respond rapidly (seconds) and are sufficiently fast to detect small oscillations in blood gases associated with breathing. The mechanisms by which changes in P_{CO_2}, pH and P_{O_2} are detected are not fully understood, but are believed to involve inhibition of K^+ channels in the glomus cell, with consequent depolarization, Ca^{2+} entry and release of neurotransmitters in the dense granules.

Adaptation: chronic respiratory disease and altitude

When hypercapnia (raised arterial P_{CO_2}) is prolonged, for example in chronic respiratory disease, CSF pH gradually returns to normal due to an adaptive and compensatory increase in HCO_3^- transport across the blood–brain barrier. The drive to breathe from the central chemoreceptor is consequently reduced, even though P_{CO_2} is still high. Associated with this, there is occasionally a loss of sensitivity to further increases in $P_{a_{CO_2}}$, and the patient's ventilation is then primarily controlled by the level of P_{O_2} (**hypoxic drive**). Care must be taken with such patients, as giving high concentrations of O_2 in order to increase blood O_2 saturation may raise the P_{O_2} sufficiently to depress the hypoxic drive and hence ventilation. Normally, approximately 23–28% O_2 is given to such patients. This leads to a sufficiently small rise in $P_{a_{O_2}}$ as to have little effect on the hypoxic drive, but because of the steep slope of the O_2 dissociation curve (Chapter 8), it can result in a significant improvement in O_2 content. At high altitudes, ventilation is stimulated by the low atmospheric P_{O_2}. This leads to **hypocapnia** and alkalosis (as more CO_2 is blown off), which depress ventilation. Over some days, the pH of CSF returns to normal due to HCO_3^- transport out of the CSF, even though the P_{CO_2} remains low, and consequently ventilation increases again. Over a longer period, blood pH returns to normal due to renal compensation (Chapter 10). These processes form part of the **acclimatization to altitude**.

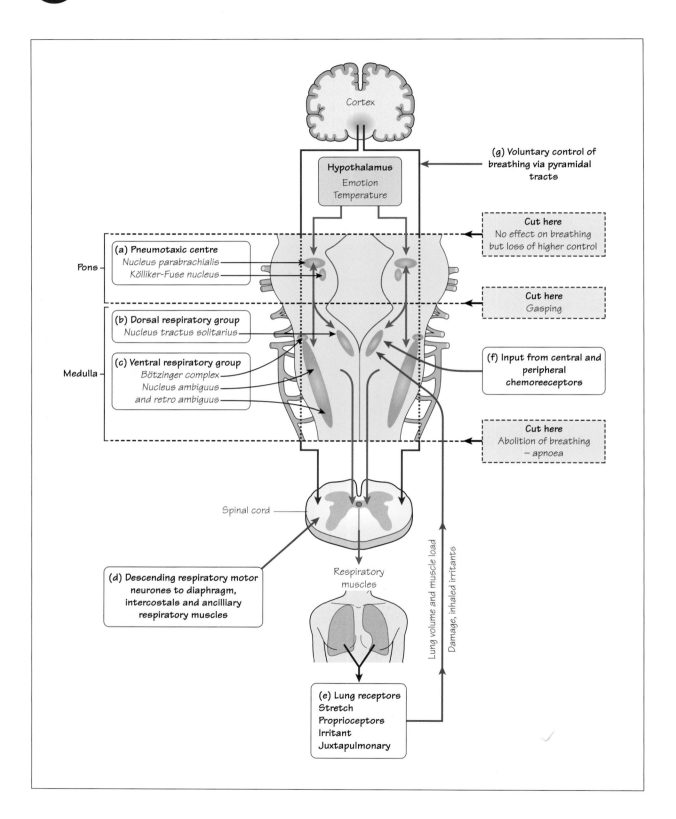

Control of breathing involves a **central pattern generator** in the brainstem that sets the basic rhythm and pattern of ventilation and controls the respiratory muscles. It is modulated by higher centres and feedback from **sensors**, including **chemoreceptors** (Chapter 11) and lung **mechanoreceptors**. The neural networks involved are complex, reflecting the need to coordinate ventilation with functions such as coughing, swallowing and vocalization.

Brainstem and central pattern generator

The **central pattern generator** determines the rate and pattern of breathing, and is a complex network encompassing diffuse groups of respiratory neurones in the **pons** and **medulla**. These contain **inspiratory** and **expiratory** neurones, with activity corresponding to inspiration and expiration, although others show more complex relationships. **Reciprocal inhibition** means activity of inspiratory neurones inhibits activity of expiratory neurones, and vice versa.

The **medulla** contains two groups of respiratory neurones. The **dorsal respiratory group** (DRG; Fig. 12b) in the **nucleus tractus solitarii** contains inspiratory neurones and receives ascending input from central and peripheral chemoreceptors (Chapter 11; Fig. 12f), and from lung receptors via the vagus (Fig. 12e). The ventrolateral medulla contains a column of neurones extending from the lateral reticular nucleus and through the **nucleus ambiguus**, comprising the **caudal** (expiratory neurones) and **rostral** (inspiratory neurones) **ventral respiratory groups** (VRG) and **pre-Bötzinger** and **Bötzinger** complexes (Fig. 12c). Although the pre-Bötzinger complex contains neurones with intrinsic activity (pacemakers), these may only be associated with **gasping**, an autoresuscitative mechanism following hypoxia, as sectioning between the medulla and pons tends to abolish eupnoea (normal breathing) and lead to gasping in the absence of vagal input. Descending output from the medulla regulates activity of respiratory muscle motor neurones (intercostals, phrenic (diaphragm), abdominal) (Fig. 12d).

The **pneumotaxic centre** is located in the **nucleus parabrachialis** and **Kölliker–Fuse nucleus** of the **pons** (Fig. 12a), and has a critical role in eupnoea and mediating responses to lung receptor stimulation (see below). It receives ascending input from the VRG, although vagal input from lung stretch receptors is routed via the DRG. The input from stretch receptors is important for timing of respiratory rhythm and especially switching inspiration off as lung volume increases. In the absence of vagal input, sectioning the mid-pons causes **apneusis** (prolonged inspiratory effort with short expirations); it has therefore been suggested that there is an **apneustic centre** in the caudal pons, possibly associated with Kölliker–Fuse nucleus. Descending input from the hypothalamus and higher centres mediates the effects of factors such as emotion and temperature on breathing, but eupnoea is maintained following sectioning above the pons (Fig. 12), although voluntary control is lost. Voluntary control of breathing is mediated by motor neurones from the cortex contained in the **pyramidal tracts**, which bypass the pneumotaxic and medullary respiratory areas (Fig. 12g). Certain rare brainstem lesions can leave the voluntary pathways intact while impairing brainstem mechanisms, so ventilation may cease when the patient falls asleep (*Ondine's curse*; Chapter 44).

The **origin of the respiratory rhythm** is controversial. Whereas some place this in the VRG and pre-Bötzinger complex, others suggest a *switching concept*, with eupnoea reflecting the output of a pontomedullary neuronal circuit that includes pneumotaxic (and apneustic) centres, VRG and DRG. In either case, cycling or switching due to reciprocal inhibition and 'off switches' within these networks is probably the source of the rhythm of breathing rather than specific pacemaker neurones.

Lung receptors and reflexes

Stretch receptors are located in smooth muscle of the bronchial walls. These are mostly **slowly adapting** (continue to fire with sustained stimulation). Their afferent nerves ascend via the vagus. Stimulation of stretch receptors causes inspiration to be shorter and shallower and delays the next cycle. These receptors are largely responsible for the **Hering–Breuer inspiratory reflex**, where lung inflation inhibits inspiratory muscle activity. Conversely, the **deflation reflex** augments inspiratory muscle activity on lung deflation. These reflexes are weak during normal breathing in adults, but become more relevant when tidal volume is large (>1 L, e.g. in exercise). The reflex is very sensitive in neonates to protect the lungs against overinflation due to the highly compliant nature of the chest wall.

Juxtapulmonary or 'J' receptors are located on alveolar and bronchial walls, close to the capillaries. Their afferents are small unmyelinated (C-fibre) or myelinated nerves in the vagus. Activation causes **apnoea** (cessation of breathing) or rapid shallow breathing, falls in heart rate and blood pressure, laryngeal constriction and relaxation of skeletal muscles. J receptors are stimulated by increased alveolar wall fluid, pulmonary congestion and oedema, microembolisms and inflammatory mediators such as histamine – all of which are associated with lung disease. The general action of J receptors is depression of somatic and visceral activity, which may be appropriate for serious lung damage as this would suppress metabolism in the face of compromised gas exchange.

Irritant receptors are located throughout airways between epithelial cells, with rapidly adapting afferent myelinated fibres in the vagus. Receptors in the trachea lead to cough – those in lower airways to hyperpnoea. They also cause reflex bronchial and laryngeal constrictions. Irritant receptors are stimulated by irritant gases, smoke and dust (Chapters 18 and 33), but also by rapid large inflations and deflations, airway deformation, pulmonary congestion and inflammation. Irritant receptors are responsible for the deep augmented breaths or sighs seen every 5–20 minutes at rest, which reverse the slow collapse of the lungs that occurs in quiet breathing. They may be involved with the first deep gasps of the newborn ('first breath') and the Hering–Breuer deflationary reflex.

Proprioceptors (position/length sensors) are located in the Golgi tendon organs, muscle spindles and joints of the respiratory muscles, but not diaphragm. Afferents lead to the spinal cord via dorsal roots, stimulated by shortening and load in respiratory muscles, although not diaphragm. They are important for coping with increased load and achieving optimal tidal volume and frequency. Input from non-respiratory muscles and joints can also stimulate breathing, for example during exercise.

Other receptors that may modulate respiration:

Pain receptors: stimulation often causes brief apnoea followed by increased breathing.

Receptors in the *trigeminal region* and *larynx*: stimulation may give rise to apnoea or laryngeal spasm.

Arterial baroreceptors: stimulation depresses breathing.

13 Pulmonary circulation and anatomical right-to-left shunts

(a) Pulmonary and systemic circulation and normal anatomical right-to-left shunts

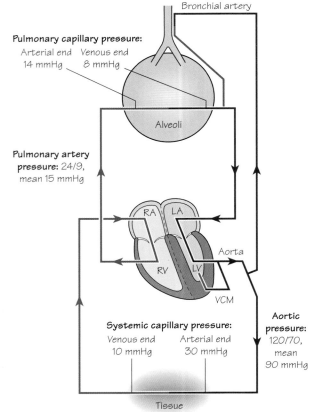

Bronchial artery

Pulmonary capillary pressure:
Arterial end   Venous end
14 mmHg   8 mmHg

Alveoli

Pulmonary artery pressure: 24/9, mean 15 mmHg

RA   LA

Aorta

RV   LV

VCM

Systemic capillary pressure:
Venous end   Arterial end
10 mmHg   30 mmHg

Aortic pressure: 120/70, mean 90 mmHg

Tissue

VCM = venae cordis minimae (thebesian veins)

(b) The initial effects of a 20% right-to-left shunt on arterial O_2 and CO_2 contents and partial pressures

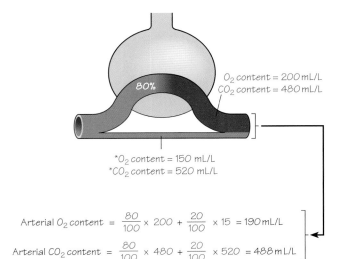

80%

O_2 content = 200 mL/L
CO_2 content = 480 mL/L

*O_2 content = 150 mL/L
*CO_2 content = 520 mL/L

$$\text{Arterial } O_2 \text{ content } = \frac{80}{100} \times 200 + \frac{20}{100} \times 15 = 190\,\text{mL/L}$$

$$\text{Arterial } CO_2 \text{ content } = \frac{80}{100} \times 480 + \frac{20}{100} \times 520 = 488\,\text{mL/L}$$

*Note: The mixed venous contents used are normal values. In fact, the abnormal arterial contents would lead to abnormal mixed venous contents so this simple analysis underestimates the effects on arterial contents.

The P_{O_2} and P_{CO_2} that result from these O_2 and CO_2 contents can be found from the O_2 and CO_2 dissociation curves:

● ■ Normal O_2 and CO_2 pressures and contents

○ □ O_2 and CO_2 pressures and contents following mixing 20% mixed venous blood with 80% blood undergoing normal gas exchange

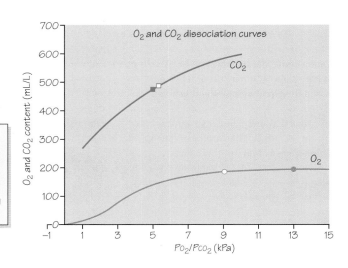

O_2 and CO_2 dissociation curves

CO_2

O_2

O_2 and CO_2 content (mL/L)

P_{O_2}/P_{CO_2} (kPa)

Pulmonary circulation compared with the systemic circulation (Fig. 13a)

The **pulmonary circulation** is in series with the **systemic circulation**, and pulmonary blood flow nearly equals aortic blood flow. **Pulmonary vascular resistance** is only about one-sixth of systemic resistance, and the thin-walled right ventricle needs only to generate a mean **pulmonary artery pressure** of about 15 mmHg to drive the cardiac output through the lungs. Systemic pressures are higher (Fig. 13a), dropping steeply across the main resistance vessel, the arteriole, to give a capillary flow which is usually non-pulsatile. Pulmonary vascular resistance is more evenly distributed in the microcirculation and pulmonary capillary flow remains pulsatile.

Local systemic resistance and blood flow are controlled by sympathetic nerves, metabolites and other substances acting on arterioles. Both sympathetic and parasympathetic nerves innervate pulmonary vessels, but their influence is weak in most circumstances. Systemic arterioles dilate in response to hypoxia, increasing flow and hence oxygen delivery to hypoxic tissues. In contrast, **hypoxic pulmonary vasoconstriction** occurs in the pulmonary circulation. This response, which is accentuated by high P_{CO_2}, improves gas exchange by diverting blood from underventilated to well-ventilated regions (Chapter 14). The response is unhelpful in the presence of global lung hypoxia, at altitude or in respiratory failure, where it may contribute to the development of pulmonary hypertension and right-sided heart failure.

Systemic vascular beds (especially the renal and cerebral) respond to changes in perfusion pressure by constricting or dilating to hold blood flow fairly constant. This **autoregulation** does not occur in the pulmonary circulation. As cardiac output increases in exercise, pulmonary vascular resistance falls, as vessels are recruited and distended and the rise in pulmonary arterial pressure is small. The pulmonary circulation acts as a blood reservoir and the volume it contains varies, being about 450 mL when upright and 800 mL when lying down. Inspiration also increases pulmonary vascular volume.

Fluid balance across capillaries is determined by hydrostatic and oncotic pressures (the **Starling forces**; see *The Cardiovascular System at a Glance*) across capillary walls. **Capillary oncotic pressure** opposes filtration and is about 27 mmHg in both circulations. Although hydrostatic pressure is low in the pulmonary capillaries ($\sim$10 mmHg), net filtration of fluid occurs in pulmonary capillaries as it does in systemic capillaries. Other factors favouring filtration are **interstitial oncotic pressure**, which is relatively high in the lungs (about 18 mmHg) and **interstitial hydrostatic pressure**, which is negative (about -4 mmHg). **Pulmonary oedema** occurs when these forces are altered to increase net filtration above the rate that can be cleared by the pulmonary lymphatics. For example, it may occur when pulmonary capillary pressure is increased in **mitral stenosis** and **left ventricular failure**. **Inspiratory crepitations** (crackles) on auscultation in these conditions are probably caused by popping open of airways in lungs stiffened by congestion with blood. They are most obvious at the bases, where hydrostatic pressure is highest. Pulmonary congestion and oedema (and hence breathlessness in these conditions) are worsened by the increase in pulmonary blood volume lying down.

Anatomical or true right-to-left shunts

Ideally, all venous blood emerging from tissues would return to the right side of the heart to be pumped through the gas-exchanging lung. In fact, part of the blood draining the **bronchial circulation** joins the pulmonary vein. This part results in deoxygenated blood from the airways contaminating blood returning from alveoli (Fig. 13a). In addition, a small amount of the coronary venous blood drains directly into the left ventricular cavity via the **venae cordis minimae (Thebesian veins)**. These additions of deoxygenated (right-sided) blood to oxygenated (left-sided) blood are known as anatomical **right-to-left shunts**. In healthy people, they are equivalent to 2% or less of the cardiac output, but they explain why arterial P_{O_2} is less than alveolar P_{O_2} even though pulmonary capillary blood equilibrates with alveolar gas.

In disease, right-to-left shunting of blood may be much larger. **Atelectasis** (airless lung) or **consolidation** in **pneumonia** will result in pulmonary arterial blood supplying the affected region failing to undergo gas exchange. Right-to-left shunts are also the cause of reduced arterial oxygenation in **cyanotic congenital heart disease** such as **tetralogy of Fallot**. Atrial or ventricular septal defects do not usually cause impaired gas exchange and cyanosis, as the higher left-sided pressures give rise to **left-to-right shunts** in which some oxygenated blood is pumped again through the lungs. If a large left-to-right shunt remains untreated, eventually the excessive pulmonary blood flow leads to pulmonary hypertension. As right ventricular pressure increases, the shunt through the atrial or ventricular septal defect may then reverse to give a right-to-left shunt and cyanosis (Eisenmenger's syndrome).

Effect of right-to-left shunts on arterial blood gases

In the right-to-left shunt, shown schematically in Fig. 13b, 20% of blood fails to pass through functioning alveoli and its O_2 and CO_2 contents remain at mixed venous levels of 150 and 520 mL/L, respectively. Eighty per cent of the blood undergoes normal gas exchange, emerging with normal O_2 and CO_2 contents of 200 and 480 mL/L, respectively. The initial effect on arterial gas contents is calculated from a weighted average of the contents in these two bloodstreams. This gives an arterial O_2 content 10 mL/L below normal and CO_2 content 8 mL/L above normal. From the flat part of the oxygen dissociation curve, it can be seen that the resulting arterial P_{O_2} is about 9 kPa (68 mmHg) compared with the normal 13 kPa (97 mmHg). The much steeper CO_2 dissociation curve means the rise in P_{CO_2} is small, from the normal value of 5.3 kPa (40 mmHg) to about 5.5 kPa (41 mmHg).

If the respiratory system is otherwise normal, the reduced P_aO_2 and increased P_aCO_2 simulate ventilation via the chemoreceptors and the CO_2 washed-out of the functioning areas restores arterial CO_2 content and P_aCO_2 to normal. In contrast, increased ventilation has little effect on arterial oxygen content and P_{O_2}, as blood draining the ventilated areas of the lung was already saturated. If hypoxia is severe, the stimulation in ventilation is often great enough to reduce P_aCO_2 below normal. Typically, in a right-to-left shunt, there is a low P_aO_2 with a normal or low P_aCO_2.

(a) Different types of V_A/Q regions

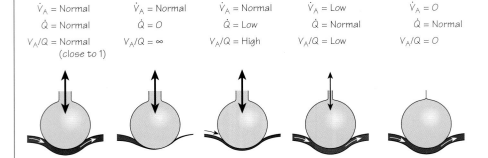

Normal	Dead space	Dead-space effect	Shunt effect	True/anatomical shunt
$\dot{V}_A$ = Normal	$\dot{V}_A$ = Normal	$\dot{V}_A$ = Normal	$\dot{V}_A$ = Low	$\dot{V}_A$ = 0
$\dot{Q}$ = Normal	$\dot{Q}$ = 0	$\dot{Q}$ = Low	$\dot{Q}$ = Normal	$\dot{Q}$ = Normal
V_A/Q = Normal (close to 1)	V_A/Q = ∞	V_A/Q = High	V_A/Q = Low	V_A/Q = 0

(b) Variation of ventilation, $\dot{V}_A$, perfusion, $\dot{Q}$ and ventilation–perfusion ratio, V_A/Q with vertical height in the upright lung

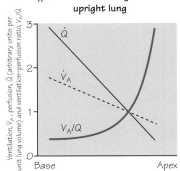

Po_2 and O_2 contents of blood from these regions breathing air and oxygen

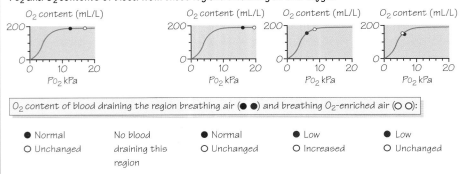

O_2 content of blood draining the region breathing air (● ●) and breathing O_2-enriched air (O O):

● Normal	No blood draining this region	● Normal	● Low	● Low
O Unchanged		O Unchanged	O Increased	O Unchanged

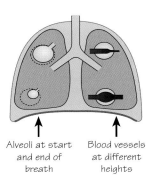

Alveoli at start and end of breath

Blood vessels at different heights

(c) The effect of a mixture of high and low V_A/Q regions on arterial blood gases

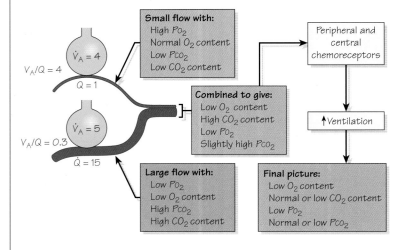

$\dot{V}_A$ = 4
V_A/Q = 4
Q = 1

Small flow with:
High Po_2
Normal O_2 content
Low Pco_2
Low CO_2 content

Peripheral and central chemoreceptors

Combined to give:
Low O_2 content
High CO_2 content
Low Po_2
Slightly high Pco_2

↑ Ventilation

$\dot{V}_A$ = 5
V_A/Q = 0.3
$\dot{Q}$ = 15

Large flow with:
Low Po_2
Low O_2 content
High Pco_2
High CO_2 content

Final picture:
Low O_2 content
Normal or low CO_2 content
Low Po_2
Normal or low Pco_2

(d) Alveolar air equation

This predicts the Po_2 in the functioning or 'ideal' alveoli

$$P_{A}O_2 \cong P_IO_2 - \frac{P_aco_2}{R}$$

R = The respiratory gas exchange ratio = $\dfrac{CO_2 \text{ production}}{O_2 \text{ consumption}}$

(R is usually about 0.8)

P_Io_2 = Inspired O_2 partial pressure
P_aco_2 = Arterial CO_2 partial pressure (≈ alveolar)

At rest, alveolar ventilation and pulmonary blood flow are similar, each being around 5 L/min. Ventilation ($\dot{V}_A$) and perfusion ($\dot{Q}$) may vary in different lung regions, but for optimal gas exchange they must be matched. Areas with high perfusion need high ventilation, and, ideally, local ventilation–perfusion ratios (V_A/Q) should be close to 1. Ventilation–perfusion mismatching or inequality is said to occur when regional V_A/Q ratios vary, with many being much greater or less than 1 (Fig. 14a). A right-to-left shunt from complete collapse or consolidation of a region (Chapter 13) has $V_A/Q = 0$, and can be viewed as an extreme example of ventilation–perfusion mismatching. At the other extreme, alveolar dead space from a pulmonary embolus is a ventilated region without perfusion and $V_A/Q = \infty$. Regions where V_A/Q is much greater than 1 have excessive ventilation or **dead-space effect** and blood from them has a high P_{O_2} and a low P_{CO_2}. Regions with V_A/Q much less than 1 behave qualitatively like shunts and are sources of **shunt effect** or **venous admixture**. Blood draining them has undergone some gas exchange, but P_{O_2} is lower and P_{CO_2} higher than normal. The effect on P_{O_2} and O_2 content draining different V_A/Q regions both during air breathing and during oxygen breathing is shown in Fig. 14a (lower panel).

Effect of the upright posture on perfusion, ventilation and V_A/Q (Fig. 14b)

Hydrostatic pressure in all vessels varies with vertical height above or below the heart because of the weight of blood. On standing, the increased pressure at the lung bases distends vessels, increasing flow. Pressures generated by the right side of the heart are low, and higher up the lung vascular pressures in diastole may fall below alveolar pressure at the venous end of the pulmonary capillary. In such regions, flow is reduced and determined by the difference between arterial and alveolar pressure. There may be regions at the apices – especially in haemorrhage or positive-pressure ventilation – where alveolar pressure also exceeds pressure at the arterial end of the pulmonary capillaries. The vessels collapse completely for part of each cardiac cycle, giving low intermittent flow. The net result is a blood flow per unit volume of lung tissue that falls progressively from base to apex.

Gravity also affects intrapleural pressure, which is less negative at the base than at the apex. As a result, at functional residual capacity, apical alveoli are more expanded – with less capacity for further expansion during inspiration – than at the bases. Consequently, ventilation is also higher at the base than at the apex. The effect of gravity on ventilation is less marked than on perfusion and so V_A/Q is higher at the apex than at the base. In young people, the degree of mismatching is modest and has little effect on blood gases because the regions with low VA/Q are still ventilated enough to nearly saturate the blood passing through them with oxygen. The scatter of ventilation–perfusion ratios increases with age and contributes to the reduction in P_aO_2 seen in the elderly.

Ventilation–perfusion matching in disease

Increased ventilation–perfusion mismatching is an important cause of gas exchange problems in many respiratory diseases, including asthma, chronic obstructive pulmonary disease (COPD), pneumonia and pulmonary oedema. Regions of low V_A/Q may arise when airways are partly blocked by bronchoconstriction, inflammation or secretions and high V_A/Q areas arise in emphysematous areas where capillaries are lost or pulmonary emboli are partially blocking blood flow. **Hypoxic vasoconstriction** (Chapter 13) helps reduce the severity of ventilation–perfusion mismatching by diverting blood from regions with low V_A/Q to regions that are better ventilated.

Effect of ventilation–perfusion mismatching on arterial blood gases

Blood emerging from areas with high V_A/Q might be expected to compensate for blood from areas with low V_A/Q. This is not the case, for two reasons (Fig. 14c). First, although P_{O_2} will be increased in high V_A/Q regions, oxygen content is raised little, as blood is normally nearly saturated. Blood draining regions with low V_A/Q and low P_{O_2} (especially if <8 kPa, 60 mmHg) will have significantly reduced oxygen content. In addition, these areas contribute more blood than areas with high V_A/Q, which are typically caused by reduced perfusion. The net effect of mixing blood from areas with a wide range of ventilation–perfusion ratios is a low arterial O_2 content and P_aO_2. CO_2 content is less severely affected because the overventilated areas do lose extra CO_2 and partly compensate for low V_A/Q regions. Moreover, any abnormalities of P_aO_2 and P_aCO_2 will lead to a reflex increase in ventilation, which usually corrects or overcorrects the raised P_aCO_2 while being less effective at raising P_aO_2. The final arterial blood gas picture, a low P_aO_2 and a normal or low P_aCO_2, is similar to that resulting from anatomical right-to-left shunts (Chapter 13).

One difference is that arterial hypoxia caused by ventilation–perfusion mismatching improves much more with oxygen therapy than that caused by a shunt. In a hypoxic patient with a pure shunt, the **oxygen-enriched air** fails to reach the shunted blood. In V_A/Q mismatching, increased oxygen fraction can increase local P_{O_2} in areas of low V_A/Q (Fig. 14a), giving rise to significant improvement in arterial oxygen content and pressure.

Assessment of ventilation–perfusion mismatching

Regional ventilation and perfusion can be visualized by inhalation and infusion of appropriate radioisotopes (Chapter 21). A simple but useful index of the degree of mismatching is the difference between P_{O_2} in gas-exchanging or 'ideal' alveoli and in arterial blood. Ideal alveolar P_{O_2} can be calculated from the **alveolar air equation** (Fig. 14d). An increased **A–a P_{O_2} gradient** (A = alveolar P_{O_2}, a = arterial P_{O_2}) is usually caused by ventilation–perfusion mismatching or anatomical right-to-left shunts. In healthy young people, there is a small A–a gradient (<2 kPa) arising from the normal anatomical right-to-left shunts, discussed in Chapter 13. The normal value for A–a gradient increases with age and in a healthy 80-year-old may be as high as 5 kPa (38 mmHg).

Table 1

Typical values in a healthy but sedentary 20-year-old man at rest and in max. exercise

	Rest	Maximal exercise
Heart rate (bpm)	70	200
Stroke volume (mL)	75	90
Cardiac output (mL/min)	5 250	18 000
Arterial–mixed venous O_2 content* (mL/mL)	0.048	0.167
O_2 consumption (mL/min)	250	3 000
Ventilation (mL/min)	7 500	140 000
Respiratory frequency (breaths/min)	15	56
Tidal volume (mL)	500	2 500

(*= O_2 extraction)

(b) Typical alveolar ventilation, P_{CO_2} and P_{O_2}, at altitudes between sea level (0 m) and 6000 m for subjects exposed acutely (red solid line) and chronically (blue solid line) following acclimatization. The dashed line shows the values that would have occurred if alveolar ventilation remained at its sea level value.

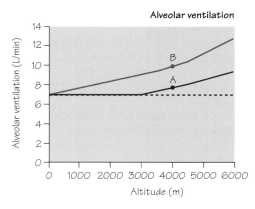

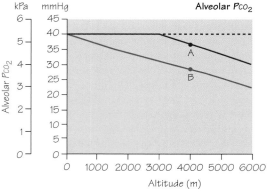

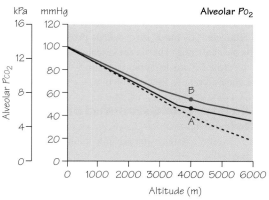

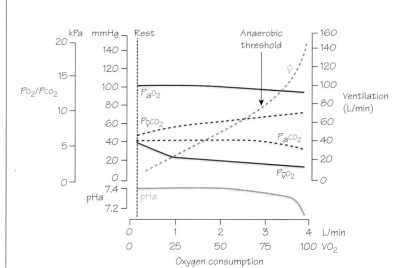

(a) Typical changes in ventilation $\dot{V}$, arterial P_{O_2} (P_aO_2), arterial P_{CO_2} (P_aCO_2), arterial pH (pHa), mixed venous P_{O_2} (P_vO_2) and mixed venous P_{CO_2} (P_vCO_2) in a fit young man as oxygen consumption is increased from its resting value of 0.25 L/min to his maximum oxygen consumption of 4 L/min.

Exercise

Resting arterial oxygen saturation is close to 100% and oxygen content cannot be raised significantly during exercise. **Oxygen delivery** (arterial oxygen content × blood flow) to exercising muscle is increased by increasing muscle blood flow, made possible by metabolic vasodilatation. **Oxygen extraction** from the delivered blood is also increased.

For the whole body, **oxygen consumption** (mL/min) = cardiac output (mL/min) × (arterial–mixed venous oxygen content) (mL/mL). In active muscle, oxygen unloading from haemoglobin is aided by the reduced tissue P_{O_2} and the rightward shift of the oxyhaemoglobin dissociation curve caused by local increases in P_{CO_2}, $[H^+]$ and temperature. Maximum oxygen extraction does not vary greatly with fitness, and the main factor determining **maximum oxygen consumption ($\dot{V}O_2$ max)** is the maximum cardiac output. $\dot{V}O_2$ max is an index of fitness and in a young man this might be 12 times resting oxygen consumption (Table 1) and more in an athlete.

In exercise, mixed venous blood has a reduced P_{O_2} and increased P_{CO_2}. As blood passes through the pulmonary capillaries, the increased alveolar to blood partial pressure gradients increase O_2 uptake and CO_2 output. In mild to moderate exercise, alveolar ventilation is accurately matched to metabolism and P_aO_2, P_aCO_2 and arterial pH (pHa) are maintained at resting values (Fig. 15a). The mechanisms initiating and controlling the ventilatory response remain uncertain. In heavy exercise, increased anaerobic metabolism increases lactic acid production and reduces arterial pH. This gives an extra stimulus to breathing via the peripheral chemoreceptors, and at this **anaerobic threshold** the relationship between ventilation and oxygen consumption becomes steeper and P_aCO_2 falls (Fig. 15a).

Exercise intolerance is a common symptom of many diseases, and the inability to raise the cardiac output adequately is the main underlying mechanism in many diseases. In anaemia oxygen delivery to the muscles is reduced because of reduce arterial oxygen content. In some respiratory diseases, limited ability to increase ventilation or incomplete equilibrium in the pulmonary capillary may limit exercise.

Altitude

Barometric pressure falls progressively with increasing altitude from about 101 kPa (760 mmHg) at sea level to 33.6 kPa (252 mmHg) on the summit of Everest (see Chapter 4), but oxygen fraction remains constant at 0.209. Moist inspired P_{O_2} ($0.209 \times (P_B - P_{H2O})$) is about 19.9 kPa (149 mmHg) at sea level and about 5.7 kPa (43 mmHg) on the summit of Everest.

If ventilation remains unchanged, reduced inspired P_{O_2} inevitably leads to reduced P_aO_2 but P_aCO_2 ($\propto CO_2$ production/alveolar ventilation) will be unaltered. This is the situation initially when a person ascends to altitudes up to about 3000 m (9840 ft) (Fig. 15b). Hypoxic carotid body chemoreceptor stimulation occurs, but any ventilatory increase lowers P_aCO_2, which depresses ventilation. Above 3000 m the more severe hypoxia does increase ventilation and P_aCO_2 falls (Fig. 15b). **Acute mountain sickness** commonly develops some hours after rapid ascent to altitudes above 3600 m (12 000 ft) with symptoms such as fatigue, nausea, anorexia, dizziness, headaches and sleep disturbance. It can progress to life-threatening **high-altitude pulmonary oedema** and/or **high-altitude cerebral oedema**, which usually require immediate descent. The more benign symptoms improve with time, a process known as **acclimatization**. Over the next few days, ventilation increases, raising P_aO_2 and lowering P_aCO_2 (A to B, Fig. 15b). During this period the initial alkalosis of arterial blood and cerebrospinal fluid (CSF) is corrected by bicarbonate transport out of the CSF and renal bicarbonate excretion. A gradual normalization of arterial and CSF pH was originally thought to explain the gradual increase of ventilation, but other mechanisms, such as increased sensitivity of the peripheral chemoreceptors to hypoxia and changes in the central nervous system reflex pathways, are also important. **Erythropoietin** production by the kidney is stimulated by hypoxia, and haemoglobin concentration rises from 150 g/L to around 200 g/L after a few weeks at high altitude, aiding acclimatization by increasing arterial oxygen content.

At altitude the concentration of **2,3-diphosphoglycerate** in red blood cells increases and P_aCO_2 falls, and they cause opposite shifts (right and left respectively) of the oxyhaemoglobin dissociation curve, which at many altitudes results in little net change in oxygen affinity. At very high altitude the very low P_aCO_2 shifts the curve to the left and the beneficial effect of increased oxygen binding in the lungs outweighs the impaired oxygen release in the tissues.

With acclimatization humans can live at much higher altitudes than it is possible to tolerate acutely. The highest long-term human settlement was Quilcha, Chilie (5334 m, 17 500 ft), from where miners walked to work at the Aucanquilcha mine 610 m (2000 ft) higher. Sudden exposure to the summit of Everest would cause a healthy sea level dweller to lose consciousness in less than 2 minutes but a few very fit and fully acclimatized people have climbed it without supplementary oxygen.

The hypoxic pulmonary vasoconstriction that aids ventilation–perfusion matching at sea level causes an unhelpful global vasoconstriction at high altitude. In some people living above 2500 m (8200 ft) this becomes excessive, leading to pulmonary hypertension and right ventricular failure. Excessive polycythaemia also often occurs in these patients, contributing to this **chronic mountain sickness (Monge's disease)**.

Diving

Diving into water affects the respiratory system in many ways. Breath-hold diving initiates several reflexes, leading to the cardiovascular and respiratory effects of the **diving response**. Immersion of the face in water stimulates receptors around the eyes and nose supplied by the trigeminal nerves, leading to reflex apnoea, bradycardia and widespread vasoconstriction. The apnoea helps prevent water inhalation. The oxygen-conserving bradycardia and vasoconstriction are enhanced by reflexes from the carotid body chemoreceptors but antagonized by reflexes from lung stretch receptors. The cardiovascular responses are usually modest in humans, but excessive bradycardia sometimes occurs, especially following unexpected immersion during expiration, and this may explain some accidental deaths in water.

The weight of the water increases the pressure on the body by 1 atmosphere (101 kPa, 760 mmHg) for every 10 m (33 ft) below the surface. Even 1 m below the surface breathing through a snorkel becomes difficult because the pressure on the chest opposes inspiration. In **SCUBA diving** greater depths are made possible by pressurizing the inspired, and hence alveolar gas, to ambient pressure, but this brings other problems. Using compressed air, the increased alveolar P_{N_2} raises arterial P_{N_2}, which has effects on the brain similar to alcohol intoxication and eventually leads to **nitrogen narcosis**. Dissolved nitrogen may also cause problems if the diver surfaces too rapidly. **Decompression sickness** or **the bends** occurs when the rapidly decreased pressure causes nitrogen to comes out of solution, forming bubbles in the blood and tissues, leading to musculoskeletal pains and neurological symptoms. The high pressure compresses the gas in the lungs and this expands during ascent. If the diver fails to exhale while ascending, this can rupture the lungs.

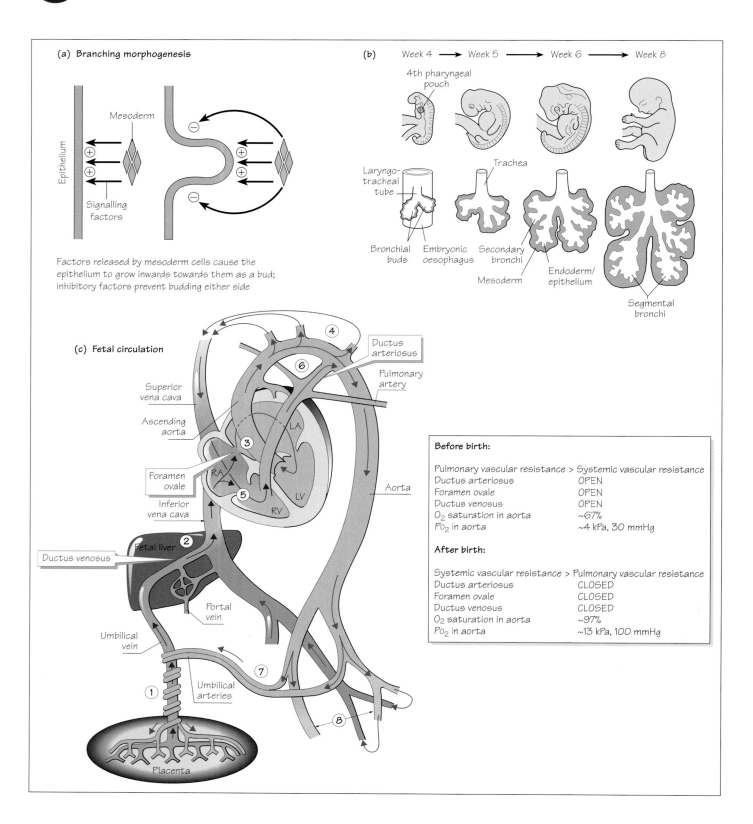

(a) Branching morphogenesis

Epithelium

Mesoderm

Signalling factors

Factors released by mesoderm cells cause the epithelium to grow inwards towards them as a bud; inhibitory factors prevent budding either side

(b) Week 4 → Week 5 → Week 6 → Week 8

4th pharyngeal pouch

Laryngo-tracheal tube

Trachea

Bronchial buds

Embryonic oesophagus

Secondary bronchi

Mesoderm

Endoderm/epithelium

Segmental bronchi

(c) Fetal circulation

Superior vena cava

Ascending aorta

Foramen ovale

Inferior vena cava

Ductus venosus

Fetal liver

Umbilical vein

Umbilical arteries

Portal vein

Placenta

Ductus arteriosus

Pulmonary artery

Aorta

LA

RA

LV

RV

Before birth:

Pulmonary vascular resistance > Systemic vascular resistance
Ductus arteriosus   OPEN
Foramen ovale   OPEN
Ductus venosus   OPEN
O_2 saturation in aorta   ~67%
Po_2 in aorta   ~4 kPa, 30 mmHg

After birth:

Systemic vascular resistance > Pulmonary vascular resistance
Ductus arteriosus   CLOSED
Foramen ovale   CLOSED
Ductus venosus   CLOSED
O_2 saturation in aorta   ~97%
Po_2 in aorta   ~13 kPa, 100 mmHg

The **embryological origins** of the lung are primitive **endoderm** of the foregut, which eventually forms the epithelium and glands of the larynx, trachea and lungs, and **splanchnic mesoderm**, which forms cartilage, smooth muscle, lung parenchyma and connective tissue. In common with many glandular organs, the lung develops by **branching morphogenesis** (Fig. 16a), with budding and branching of the endoderm/epithelium into mesoderm. The process requires reciprocal signalling between epithelium and mesoderm, with the mesoderm being primarily responsible for programming development of adjacent epithelium into the relevant structures. Many signalling molecules are vital for the orchestration of branching morphogenesis during lung development, including growth factors such as fibroblast growth factor (FGF), epidermal growth factor (EGF) and platelet-derived growth factor (PDGF); vascular endothelial growth factor (VEGF) is critical for pulmonary vascular development. Development of the respiratory system is generally divided into five stages or periods.

1. Embryonic period: The tracheobronchial tree originates from the **laryngotracheal tube**, below the fourth pharyngeal pouch at the caudal (tail) end of the primordial pharynx. The laryngotracheal tube starts to appear just prior to the fourth week of development, after the heart begins to beat. By the end of the fourth week, its end has bifurcated into two **bronchial buds**, progenitors of the two main bronchi and bronchial tree (Fig. 16b).

2. Pseudoglandular period (5–17th weeks): The bronchial buds have now developed into the primordial left and (slightly larger) right primary bronchi, which subsequently divide by branching morphogenesis into five secondary bronchi (three right, two left). At the seventh week, these have started to branch progressively into ten (right) or eight to nine (left) **segmental** (tertiary) bronchi, each of which eventually forms a **bronchopulmonary segment**. By the 17th week, most major structures of the lung have formed and are lined with columnar epithelial cells. Conducting blood vessels are present, but the gas exchange surfaces have not yet developed and fetuses delivered during this period are therefore not viable.

3. Canalicular period (16–25th weeks): Bronchial cartilage, smooth muscle, pulmonary capillaries and connective tissue develop from the mesoderm. There is progressive differentiation and thinning of epithelial cells. The bronchi will have subdivided approximately 17 times after 24 weeks, finally forming the respiratory bronchioles which themselves divide into three to six alveolar ducts and some thin-walled **terminal sacs**. These are lined by very thin **type I alveolar pneumocytes** (squamous epithelium), which together with endothelial cells from capillaries form the future **alveolocapillary membrane** (gas exchange surface). There are a few **type II alveolar pneumocytes**, secretory epithelial cells that produce surfactant. This reduces surface tension and allows expansion of the terminal sacs/alveoli (Chapter 6), but although it is present in small amounts from about the 20th week, there is insufficient to support unaided breathing until after 26 weeks (see **neonatal respiratory distress syndrome**, Chapter 17). Some gas exchange can occur at the end of this period, as there are both thin-walled terminal sacs and good vascularization, but the general level of immaturity means that fetuses born before the end of the 24th week normally die despite intensive care.

4. Saccular (terminal sac) period (24th week to parturition): Associated with rapid development in the number of terminal sacs and the pulmonary and lymphatic capillary networks. Budding from terminal sacs and walls of terminal bronchioles and thinning of type I pneumocytes lead to formation of immature alveoli from around week 32. Sufficient surfactant and vascularization are normally present between the 24 and 26th week to allow survival of some premature fetuses, although this is very variable (Chapter 17). Surfactant increases significantly in the 2 weeks before birth.

5. Alveolar period (late fetal to childhood): Clusters of immature alveoli form during the early part of this period; mature-type alveoli with thin interalveolar septa and gas exchange surfaces do not appear until after birth. **Fetal breathing** movements are present before birth, with aspiration of amniotic fluid, and these stimulate lung growth and respiratory muscle conditioning. Lung development is impaired in the absence of fetal breathing, inadequate amniotic fluid (**oligohydramnios**) or space for lung growth (Chapter 17). The increase in lung size over the first 3 years is due primarily to an increase in number of alveoli and respiratory bronchioles; thereafter, both the number and size of alveoli increase. More than 90% of alveoli are formed after birth, reaching a maximum after 7–8 years. At the end of lung development, there are approximately 23 generations of airways, with approximately 17 million branches.

Fetal circulation and birth

Gas exchange in the fetus occurs in the **placenta**. Oxygen-rich blood from the umbilical vein flows into the liver and **ductus venosus**, and thus into the vena cava. Most blood entering the right atrium is diverted into the left atrium via the **foramen ovale**; the remainder enters the right ventricle and is pumped into the pulmonary artery as in the adult (Fig. 16c). However, the vascular resistance of the pulmonary circulation is high due to the collapsed state of the lungs and vasoconstriction, and 90% of the blood is therefore shunted via the **ductus arteriosus** into the aorta (Fig. 16c). Note that the P_aO_2 in the fetus is much lower ($\sim$4 kPa, 30 mmHg) than in the adult; oxygen transport is sustained by high-affinity fetal haemoglobin (Chapter 8).

At birth, the lungs are initially 50% full of fluid which is replaced by air. During and immediately following birth, fluid is removed via the pulmonary and lymphatic circulations, and through the mouth as a result of squeezing during delivery. Expansion and filling of the alveoli with air is critically dependent on the presence of **surfactant** to lower surface tension. The initiation of gas exchange in the lungs and consequent rise in blood PO_2 cause vasodilatation of the pulmonary circulation and constriction of the ductus arteriosus, so that blood from the right side of the heart now follows its adult course via the lungs. The consequent fall in right atrial pressure causes the pressure gradient across the foramen ovale to reverse, causing functional closure within hours. The removal of venous return from the placenta also causes closure of the ductus venosus. Initially, pressure gradients keep the three fetal shunts closed, but after several months structural changes cause permanent closure. In 20% of adults this may remain incomplete for the foramen ovale, but is generally of no consequence.

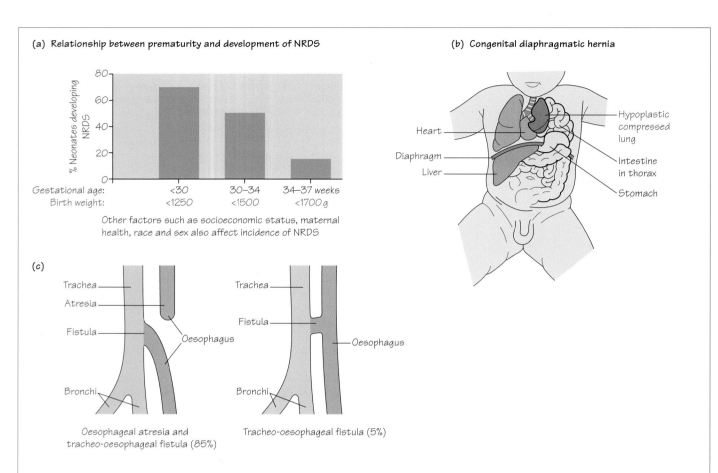

(a) Relationship between prematurity and development of NRDS

% Neonates developing NRDS

| Gestational age: | <30 | 30–34 | 34–37 weeks |
| Birth weight: | <1250 | <1500 | <1700 g |

Other factors such as socioeconomic status, maternal health, race and sex also affect incidence of NRDS

(b) Congenital diaphragmatic hernia

Heart
Diaphragm
Liver
Hypoplastic compressed lung
Intestine in thorax
Stomach

(c)

Trachea
Atresia
Fistula
Oesophagus
Bronchi

Oesophageal atresia and tracheo-oesophageal fistula (85%)

Trachea
Fistula
Oesophagus
Bronchi

Tracheo-oesophageal fistula (5%)

(d) Some genetic diseases in which the lung is a primary site of injury

Disease	Inheritance	Pathogenesis	Lung pathology
Alpha$_1$-antitrypsin deficiency	AD	Protease–antiprotease imbalance	Emphysema
Ciliary dyskinesia	AR	Impaired mucociliary clearance	Airway infection, bronchiectasis
Cystic fibrosis	AR	Abnormal chloride transport	Airway infection, bronchiectasis
Familial idiopathic fibrosis	AR	Unknown	Diffuse fibrosis
Lipoid proteinosis (Urbach–Wiethe syndrome)	AR	Lipoglycoprotein deposition in upper respiratory tract causing mucosal thickening and airway obstruction	Hyalinized or granular deposits in the tracheo-bronchial submucosa
Tracheobroncho-megaly (Mounier–Kuhn syndrome)	AR	Saccular bulges between cartilage rings resulting from atrophy of elastic and smooth muscle tissue and causing impaired mucociliary clearance	Recurrent airway infections
Congenital cartilage deficiency (Williams–Campbell syndrome)	?	Deficiency of subsegmental bronchial cartilage with airway collapse	Recurrent airway infections, bronchiectasis

AD = Autosomal dominant, AR = Autosomal recessive

Problems associated with premature birth

Neonatal respiratory distress syndrome (NRDS), otherwise known as hyaline membrane disease, occurs in approximately 2% of all births and is characterized by rapid, laboured breathing and often sternal retraction due to partial collapse of the lungs after each breath. Lung compliance is low. NRDS is most commonly caused by lack of sufficient quantities of surfactant and consequent high surface tension in the alveoli and small airways. Incidence therefore increases sharply with the degree of prematurity (Fig. 17a), although other factors may also reduce production of surfactant. When a premature birth is anticipated, the expectant mother can be treated with **corticosteroids** (betamethasone) to speed fetal lung development and surfactant production. Treatment with **exogenous surfactant** in the first 30 minutes after birth, either of natural origin or artificial, has also proved to be beneficial. Survival of neonates with NRDS often requires high positive-pressure mechanical ventilation and high levels of oxygen.

The large majority of NRDS cases are related to prematurity, with some due to other causes including damage to type II pneumocytes. A very few cases are due to a congenital absence of **pulmonary surfactant protein B**. These patients do not respond to any form of therapy and tend to die in the first few months of life.

Bronchopulmonary dysplasia (chronic lung disease of the newborn) is a long-term consequence of NRDS, primarily as a result of treatment with high positive-pressure ventilation combined with high levels of oxygen (hyperoxia). The condition is characterized by alterations in the structure and function of airways and pulmonary blood vessels, including increases in airway and vascular smooth muscle and obliteration of some microstructures. This leads to poorly reversible airway obstruction and sometimes pulmonary hypertension (high pulmonary blood pressure). Survivors may retain symptoms for many years, if not for life. There are several similarities to chronic obstructive pulmonary disease (COPD, Chapter 26) and chronic severe asthma in adults.

Several techniques have recently been designed to minimize the incidence of bronchopulmonary dysplasia in infants with NRDS. These include extracorporeal membrane oxygenation (**ECMO**), where blood is circulated via external apparatus for gas exchange; mechanical ventilation and hyperoxia are therefore not required and some success has been reported. Conversely, ECMO has not been found useful in adults with acute respiratory distress syndrome (ARDS, Chapter 41). **Partial fluid ventilation**, where the lungs are ventilated with fluids containing oxygen-carrying perfluorocarbons, has also been reported to be beneficial. Fluid ventilation circumvents problems associated with high surface tension by removing the air–liquid interface and allows small airways to open and contribute to gas exchange.

Congenital diseases

Congenital diaphragmatic hernia is the most common cause of lung hypoplasia (inadequate development of the lung), with an incidence of about one in 2000 births. Failure of the diaphragm to fuse with the membranes on the thoracic and peritoneal wall leads to a posterolateral defect, most commonly occurring on the left side (~85%), through which the abdominal viscera pass (herniate) into the thorax (Fig. 17b). This often includes the stomach, spleen and much of the intestines. The presence of the resultant mass severely restricts lung development and later inflation, leading to a significantly reduced lung volume and life-threatening breathing difficulties. The latter are the prime cause of death in congenital diaphragmatic hernia, and most infants will die because the lungs are insufficiently developed to support life outside the uterus. Although surgical correction of the defect is possible both before and after birth, the mortality rate is very high. A related but very much less common condition is **eventration of the diaphragm**, where half the diaphragm lacks adequate muscle and bulges (eventrates) into the thoracic cavity. The viscera are forced into the pocket so formed, again restricting lung development.

Tracheo-oesophageal fistula (an opening between oesophagus and trachea) is the most common abnormality of the lower respiratory tract itself, with an incidence of about one in 4000 births. Its origins are located in the fourth week of development, when the embryonic respiratory tract starts to develop and divide from the embryonic oesophagus (Chapter 16). Eighty-five per cent of cases are associated with the descending part of the oesophagus having a blind ending (**oesophageal atresia**) (Fig. 17c); the lower part of the oesophagus joins instead to the base of the trachea. As a result, normal feeding is impossible and the gut becomes distended with air. There are also consequences in utero, as normally amniotic fluid is ingested by the fetus. Thus, oesophageal atresia is commonly associated with excess amniotic fluid (**polyhydramnios**), which can lead to severe defects in the central nervous system. Some 5% of cases of tracheo-oesophageal fistula show no atresia but only a fistula, and the remainder less common variations. Rare defects involving blockage or narrowing of the trachea itself (**tracheal atresia/stenosis**) are nearly always accompanied by various types of tracheo-oesophageal fistula.

There are many **inherited disorders of haemoglobin synthesis**. In some (e.g. **thalassaemia**) there is inadequate production of the normal globin chains, and in others (e.g. HbS in **sickle cell disease**) there is production of globin chains with an abnormal amino acid sequence. They produce a variety of clinical problems mostly related to anaemia and/or alteration in the solubility (HbS) or oxygen affinity of the abnormal haemoglobin (Chapter 8).

Congenital influences on respiratory disease: several important respiratory diseases that are discussed in detail in other chapters have definite or implied genetic components, including asthma (Chapter 24), chronic obstructive pulmonary disease (Chapter 26), emphysema (Chapter 26), cystic fibrosis (Chapter 34) and pulmonary arterial hypertension (Chapter 27). Other genetically linked diseases that cause pathological problems primarily in the lung are listed in Fig. 17d.

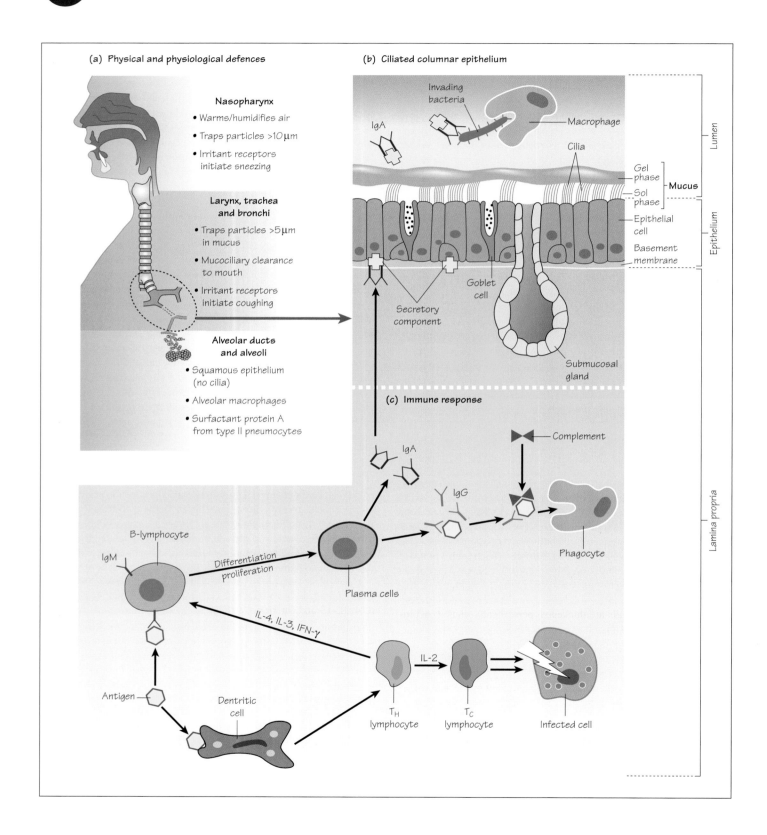

(a) Physical and physiological defences

Nasopharynx
- Warms/humidifies air
- Traps particles >10 μm
- Irritant receptors initiate sneezing

Larynx, trachea and bronchi
- Traps particles >5 μm in mucus
- Mucociliary clearance to mouth
- Irritant receptors initiate coughing

Alveolar ducts and alveoli
- Squamous epithelium (no cilia)
- Alveolar macrophages
- Surfactant protein A from type II pneumocytes

(b) Ciliated columnar epithelium

Invading bacteria

IgA

Macrophage

Cilia

Gel phase

Sol phase

Mucus

Epithelial cell

Basement membrane

Lumen

Epithelium

Goblet cell

Secretory component

Submucosal gland

(c) Immune response

IgA

Complement

IgG

Phagocyte

B-lymphocyte

IgM

Differentiation proliferation

Plasma cells

IL-4, IL-3, IFN-γ

Antigen

Dentritic cell

IL-2

T_H lymphocyte

T_C lymphocyte

Infected cell

Lamina propria

Inhalation of air also allows ingress of dust, irritant particles and pathogens. The huge surface area of the lungs provides multiple opportunities for damage, and the warm humid environment provides ideal conditions for bacterial and other infestations. The respiratory tract, however, has a range of powerful defence mechanisms. Dysfunction of these mechanisms underlies many respiratory diseases, for example asthma (Chapter 24) and fibrosis (Chapters 30 & 33).

Physical and physiological defences

The nostrils and nasopharynx provide a physical barrier to particles greater than 10 μm, in the form of hairs and mucus to which particles adhere (Fig. 18a). **Mucociliary transport** (see below) subsequently transfers these to the pharynx, where they are ingested. Only particles less than 5 μm generally get further than the trachea. The nasopharynx also provides important **humidifying** and **warming** functions for inhaled air, preventing drying of epithelium. Irritant particles in the nose and trachea, whether inhaled or transported from distal regions by mucociliary transport, stimulate irritant receptors (Chapter 12), provoking sneezing and coughing which eject foreign matter.

Mucus and airway secretions

The respiratory epithelium is covered with a 5–10 μm layer of gelatinous mucus (**gel phase**) floating on a slightly thinner fluid layer (**sol phase**) (Fig. 18b). Mucus is produced by **goblet cells** in the epithelium and **submucosal glands** (Fig. 18b). The major constituents are carbohydrate-rich glycoproteins called mucins which give mucus its gel-like nature. The fluidity and ionic composition of the sol phase are controlled by epithelial cells. The **cilia** on epithelial cells beat synchronously, and as they do so their tips catch in the gel phase and cause it to move towards the mouth, transporting particles and cellular debris with it (**mucociliary transport** or clearance). It takes approximately 40 minutes for mucus from large bronchi to reach the pharynx but several days from the respiratory bronchioles. Many factors can disrupt this mechanism, including an increase in mucus viscosity or thickness, making it harder to move (e.g. inflammation and asthma), changes in the sol phase that inhibit cilia movement or prevent attachment to the gel phase, and defects in cilia activity (**cilia dyskinesia**). Mucociliary transport is reduced by smoking, pollutants, anaesthetics and infection, and in **cystic fibrosis** dysfunctional fluid transport results in viscous mucus (Chapters 34). The rare congenital immotile cilia syndrome is due to a defective 'motor' protein in the cilia themselves. Reduced mucociliary transport causes recurrent respiratory infections that progressively damage the lungs – causing for example **bronchiectasis**, where the bronchial walls are thickened, permanently dilated and inflamed (Chapter 34 and 45).

Mucus contains several factors produced by epithelial and other cells or that are derived from plasma. A**ntiproteases** such as α_1-**antitrypsin** inhibit the action of proteases, trypsin and elastase released from bacteria and neutrophils which degrade proteins and left unchecked would damage the airways; α_1-**antitrypsin deficiency** therefore predisposes to disruption of elastin and development of emphysema (Chapter 26). **Surfactant protein A**, apart from its actions on surface tension, enhances phagocytosis by cells such as macrophages (see below) by coating or **opsonizing** (literally 'making ready to eat') bacteria and other particles. **Lysozyme** is secreted by granulocytes in large quantities in the airways and has antifungal and bactericidal properties; together with the antimicrobial proteins lactoferrin, peroxidases and neutrophil-derived defensins, it provides non-specific immunity to the respiratory tract.

Secretory immunoglobulin A (IgA) is the principal immunoglobulin in airway secretions and with IgM and IgG agglutinates and opsonizes antigenic particles; it also restricts adherence of microbes to the mucosa. Secretory IgA consists of a dimer of two IgA molecules produced by **plasma cells** (activated B lymphocytes, see below) and a glycoprotein **secretory component**. The latter is produced on the basolateral surface of epithelial cells, where it binds the IgA dimer (see Fig. 18b). The secretory IgA complex is then transferred to the luminal surface of the epithelial cell and released into the bronchial fluid (see Fig. 18b). It can account for as much as 10% of the total protein in bronchoalveolar lavage fluid. Agglutinated and opsonized antigenic particles can be subsequently ingested and removed by phagocytes such as macrophages and neutrophils.

Lung macrophages

Macrophages are mobile **mononuclear phagocytes** that are found throughout the respiratory tract. They act as sentinels in the airways, providing innate protection against inhaled microorganisms and other particles by **phagocytosis** (ingesting them) and production of potent antimicrobial agents including reactive oxygen species. Phagocytosed organic material is usually digested, whereas inorganic material is sequestered inside the cell. As alveolar epithelium does not have cilia, alveolar macrophages are key to removing material and are the major cell present in the alveoli. Other functions include clearance of surfactant proteins and suppression of unnecessary immune responses by production of **anti-inflammatory cytokines** such as interleukin-10 (IL-10) and transforming growth factor β (TGFβ). However, in more severe infections, they can initiate inflammatory responses and by release of chemoattractants such as leukotriene B_4 promote neutrophil infiltration from the plasma. They can also act as antigen-presenting cells (see below).

Basics of immunity

T and **B lymphocytes** migrate to lymph nodes, tonsils and adenoids and diffuse patches of bronchus-associated lymphoid tissue (**BALT**) within the lamina propria. Here, they interact and are programmed. Antigen is presented to **CD4+ T lymphocytes** (T helper or T_H cells) by **antigen-presenting cells**. The most important are **dendritic cells**, highly specialized mononuclear phagocytes (Fig. 18c). Macrophages, B lymphocytes and some epithelial cells can also act as antigen-presenting cells. On presentation of antigen, T_H cells release **cytokines** such as IL-2, IL-4, IL-13 and interferon-γ (IFN-γ). IL-2 activates **CD8+ T lymphocytes** (cytotoxic or T_C cells), which kill infected cells. IL-4, IL-13 and IFN-γ activate B lymphocytes in the presence of antigen binding to surface immunoglobulins (IgM) (Fig. 18c). Activated B lymphocytes proliferate and differentiate into **plasma cells** that re-enter the bloodstream. These secrete large amounts of antigen-specific antibody (immunoglobins, e.g. IgG and IgA). Binding of antibody to antigen may neutralize some toxic molecules, but more commonly activates secondary mechanisms, either directly by opsonization, allowing recognition and phagocytosis by macrophages and neutrophils, or by activation of **complement**. When activated, complement can kill pathogens by lysis (bursting the cell membrane), opsonize the antibody–antigen complex and recruit inflammatory cells. Note that allergy, for example in asthma (Chapter 24), is specifically associated with IgE, which is otherwise at low levels. For more detailed information see *Immunology at a Glance*.

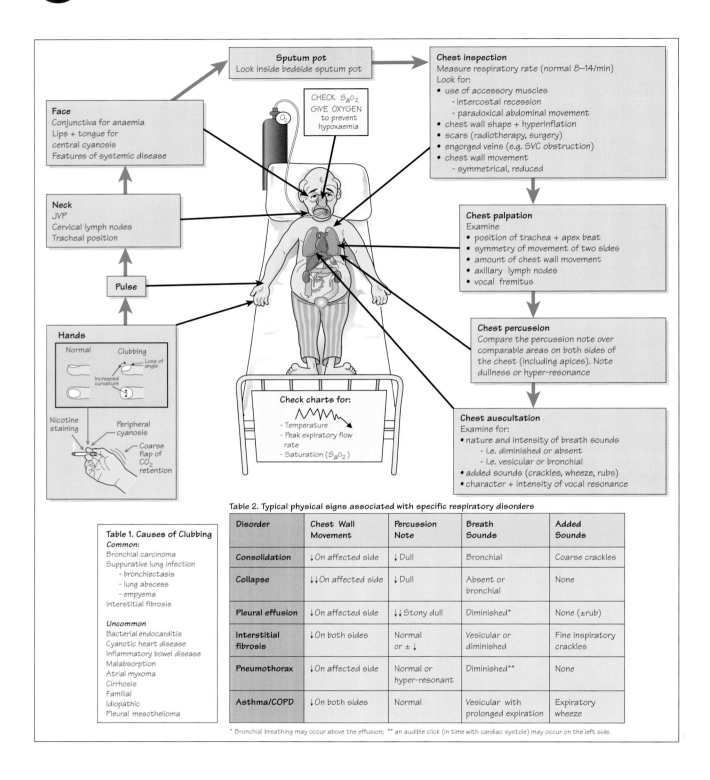

Sputum pot
Look inside bedside sputum pot

Chest inspection
Measure respiratory rate (normal 8–14/min)
Look for:
• use of accessory muscles
  - intercostal recession
  - paradoxical abdominal movement
• chest wall shape + hyperinflation
• scars (radiotherapy, surgery)
• engorged veins (e.g. SVC obstruction)
• chest wall movement
  - symmetrical, reduced

Face
Conjunctiva for anaemia
Lips + tongue for
central cyanosis
Features of systemic disease

CHECK S_aO_2
GIVE OXYGEN
to prevent
hypoxaemia

Neck
JVP
Cervical lymph nodes
Tracheal position

Chest palpation
Examine
• position of trachea + apex beat
• symmetry of movement of two sides
• amount of chest wall movement
• axillary lymph nodes
• vocal fremitus

Pulse

Hands

Normal   Clubbing

Loss of angle
Increased curvature

Nicotine staining

Peripheral cyanosis

Coarse flap of CO_2 retention

Chest percussion
Compare the percussion note over
comparable areas on both sides of
the chest (including apices). Note
dullness or hyper-resonance

Check charts for:
- Temperature
- Peak expiratory flow rate
- Saturation (S_aO_2)

Chest auscultation
Examine for:
• nature and intensity of breath sounds
  - i.e. diminished or absent
  - i.e. vesicular or bronchial
• added sounds (crackles, wheeze, rubs)
• character + intensity of vocal resonance

Table 1. Causes of Clubbing
Common:
Bronchial carcinoma
Suppurative lung infection
 - bronchiectasis
 - lung abscess
 - empyema
Interstitial fibrosis

Uncommon
Bacterial endocarditis
Cyanotic heart disease
Inflammatory bowel disease
Malabsorption
Atrial myxoma
Cirrhosis
Familial
Idiopathic
Pleural mesothelioma

Table 2. Typical physical signs associated with specific respiratory disorders

Disorder	Chest Wall Movement	Percussion Note	Breath Sounds	Added Sounds
Consolidation	↓On affected side	↓Dull	Bronchial	Coarse crackles
Collapse	↓↓On affected side	↓Dull	Absent or bronchial	None
Pleural effusion	↓On affected side	↓↓Stony dull	Diminished*	None (±rub)
Interstitial fibrosis	↓On both sides	Normal or ± ↓	Vesicular or diminished	Fine inspiratory crackles
Pneumothorax	↓On affected side	Normal or hyper-resonant	Diminished**	None
Asthma/COPD	↓On both sides	Normal	Vesicular with prolonged expiration	Expiratory wheeze

* Bronchial breathing may occur above the effusion; ** an audible click (in time with cardiac systole) may occur on the left side.

History

A comprehensive history exploring the time course, nature and severity of symptoms is the most important factor in establishing the cause of respiratory (or any other) disease. A systematic logical approach is outlined below and ensures a thorough, complete enquiry.

1 General features: age, sex, race and marital status are recorded as these may be associated with specific diseases. Thus, tuberculosis (TB) is more common in Asians, sarcoidosis in Afro-Caribbeans.

2 Presenting complaint: lists the main symptoms, usually chest pain, breathlessness, cough or haemoptysis in respiratory disease.

3 History of the presenting complaint: explores the specific features (e.g. onset and progress) of the main symptoms and associated systemic manifestations (e.g. fever, rigors, night sweats, malaise, weight loss, lymphadenopathy, arthritis and rashes). Thus, drenching night sweats and weight loss are associated with TB and cancer and erythema nodosum (inflammatory skin nodules) with sarcoidosis or TB. Obstructive sleep apnoea causes daytime sleepiness and is associated with snoring, obesity and collar size of more than 17 in. (43 cm).

- *Chest pain:* establish site, sort (pleuritic, aching), severity, onset (gradual, sudden), periodicity (intermittent, constant), duration (minutes, days), aggravating and relieving factors (i.e. worse/better with breathing, posture) and time off work. Pleuritic pain is a localized, sharp pain aggravated by deep breathing.
- *Breathlessness:* occurs at rest, on exercise or when lying flat (orthopnoea). Determine rate of onset (sudden, gradual), when it occurs (i.e. nocturnal), exercise tolerance (i.e. when walking, running or climbing stairs?) and associated symptoms (e.g. hayfever, wheeze and stridor). In chronic obstructive pulmonary disease (COPD) breathlessness is worse on exercise. In contrast, breathlessness due to pulmonary oedema may suddenly wake a sleeping (i.e. supine) patient with heart failure. Nocturnal breathlessness with wheeze or seasonal breathlessness with hayfever suggests asthma.
- *Cough:* in the morning indicates chronic bronchitis (smoker's cough), at night suggests asthma or may be persistent after viral respiratory tract infections with bronchial hyper-responsiveness. Cough may be dry or productive of sputum. In a smoker, persistent cough, change in character or a bovine cough (due to recurrent laryngeal nerve palsy) indicates development of bronchial carcinoma.
- *Sputum:* morning cough and sputum production for 3 months a year for more than 1 year defines chronic bronchitis. Yellow or green, mucopurulent sputum occurs in chest infections and when copious and foul smelling may indicate bronchiectasis. Pink frothy sputum is typical of pulmonary oedema.
- *Haemoptysis:* determine frequency and quantity (i.e. flecks in sputum, fresh red blood); more than 500 mL haemoptysis in 24 hours is life-threatening. Infection (e.g. TB, pneumonia, bronchiectasis and *Aspergillus*) accounts for approximately 80% of haemoptysis; bronchial carcinoma and rarer cause (pulmonary infarction, vasculitis) for approximately 20%.

4 Past medical history: enquire about previous respiratory conditions; childhood whooping cough is associated with adult bronchiectasis; TB may reactivate in later life. Atopy and eczema are often associated with asthma. Assess understanding of current diseases and compliance with medications. Review previous chest X-rays, hospital admissions and the need for mechanical ventilation.

5 Medications: review current and previous medications, including inhalers, nebulizers and oxygen. Determine whether recent changes are associated with new symptoms (e.g. β-blockers may precipitate or worsen asthma; cytotoxics (e.g. methotrexate) can cause pulmonary fibrosis). Record **allergies** to medications and foods.

6 Family, occupational and social history: a family history of atopy, tuberculosis, COPD or cystic fibrosis may help establish a diagnosis. **Smoking history** including duration and amount (1 pack/day for 1 year = 1 pack/year). **Alcohol abuse** predisposes to tuberculosis. **Occupation** may predispose to respiratory disease (e.g. asbestos exposure is associated with pleural plaques, fibrosis and mesothelioma; isocyanate exposure with asthma). **Environmental** factors may be important (e.g. pet birds may cause psitticosis). **Travel** is associated with specific infections (e.g. Legionnaire's disease).

Examination (Fig. 19)

Detection of typical constellations of clinical signs helps establish a diagnosis, although poor inter-observer agreement questions their reliability and emphasizes the need for other investigations.

General examination

Determine if the patient is well or unwell and whether breathing, airway and circulation are adequate. Examine breathing rate and pattern. Assess the degree of breathlessness at rest or while undressing. Check observation charts (e.g. temperature and S_aO_2) and bedside sputum pots. Note general features such as obesity, cachexia, jaundice, respiratory distress, anxiety and pain. Examine:

- *Hands:* for nicotine staining, finger clubbing (Fig. 19; Table 1), peripheral cyanosis, the fine tremor of excessive B_2-agonist therapy and the coarse tremor of a CO_2 retention flap. A 'bounding' pulse also suggests CO_2 retention.
- *Face and neck:* for lymph nodes and features of systemic diseases. Examine the conjunctiva for anaemia and the tongue (lips) for central cyanosis (blue discoloration due to an increase in deoxygenated arterial haemoglobin). Measure the jugular venous pressure (JVP) and changes with respiration (i.e. fixed and raised in superior vena cava (SVC) obstruction). Check for tracheal deviation and stridor (inspiratory wheeze due to upper airway obstruction).

Chest examination

Includes anterior and posterior inspection, palpation, percussion and auscultation, with comparison of the left and right sides. The pattern of physical signs will indicate likely diagnoses (Table 2).

- *Inspection:* includes chest and spinal shape, scars of previous radiotherapy or surgery, subcutaneous nodules, engorged chest wall veins (SVC obstruction), hyperinflation, symmetry of chest wall movement and use of accessory muscles of respiration.
- *Palpation:* examine for tenderness, apex beat position and adequate chest wall expansion (>3 cm).
- *Percussion:* assess for dullness and hyper-resonance.
- *Auscultation:* assess breath sounds and their distribution including nature (i.e. vesicular, bronchial), intensity (i.e. absent, diminished) and added sounds (wheezes, crackles, rub). **'Vesicular' breath sounds** are normal inspiratory and expiratory sounds; there is no gap between inspiration and expiration. **Bronchial breath sounds** are high-pitched ('blowing') sounds with a gap between inspiration and expiration. They occur with consolidation, collapse and above pleural effusions. Reduced breath sounds occur with effusions, consolidation, pneumothorax and raised diaphragm. **Crepitations** may be fine, fixed and inspiratory due to pulmonary fibrosis or early consolidation, or coarse due to excessive bronchial secretions (e.g. bronchiectasis). **Vocal resonance** and **tactile vocal fremitus** increase over areas of consolidation and diminish over effusions and collapsed lung.

(a) Volume–time spirograms during forced expiration from total lung capacity

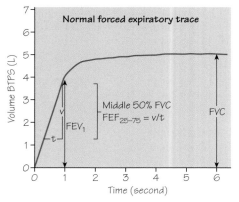

Normal forced expiratory trace

Middle 50% FVC
$FEF_{25-75} = v/t$

FEV_1

FVC

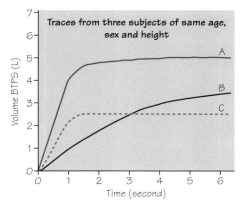

Traces from three subjects of same age, sex and height

A
B
C

FEV_1 = Forced expiratory volume in 1 second
FVC = Forced vital capacity
FEF_{25-75} = Mean forced expiratory flow from 25–75% of FVC

A = Normal respiratory system
B = Obstructive airway disease
C = Restrictive lung disease

(b) Helium dilution for measuring functional residual capacity*

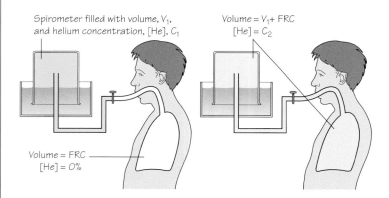

Spirometer filled with volume, V_1, and helium concentration, [He], C_1

Volume = V_1 + FRC
[He] = C_2

Volume = FRC
[He] = 0%

Starting at the end of a normal expiration (lung volume = FRC), the subject breathes in and out from the spirometer until equilibrium is reached. Since helium is poorly soluble in blood:

$$V_1 \times C_1 = (V_1 + FRC) \times C_2 \qquad \therefore FRC = V_1 \times \left(\frac{C_1 - C_2}{C_2}\right)$$

*Note: To measure TLC or RV, the subject is asked to breathe in fully or breathe out fully before breathing the helium gas mixture.

(c) The body plethysmograph for measuring lung volumes

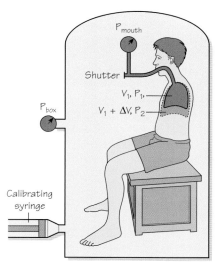

P_{mouth}

Shutter

$V_1, P_1,$
$V_1 + \Delta V, P_2$

P_{box}

Calibrating syringe

The subject inhales against a closed shutter
Lung volume expands from V_1 to $V_1 + \Delta V$
ΔV can be deduced from the rise in box pressure, P_{box} (calibrated with known volumes)
Mouth (= alveolar) pressure falls from P_1 to P_2
From Boyle's law: $V_1 \times P_1 = P_2(V_1 + \Delta V)$
Hence the original volume in the lungs, V_1, can be found

Accurate assessment of defects in airflow, lung volume or gas exchange is essential to the diagnosis and management of many respiratory disorders. It is important to note that these tests characterize 'defects'; the clinician has to diagnose 'diseases'. The normal range of many lung function tests is very wide, and it is essential to compare measured values with those predicted for the subject's age, height and sex by standard **nomograms** derived from large cross-sectional studies.

Airway resistance can be measured using a **body plethysmograph** (Chapter 7; Fig. 20c) to measure alveolar pressure. **Lung compliance** can be measured using **oesophageal pressure** to assess intrapleural pressure (for details see Chapter 6). More commonly, abnormalities of airway resistance (in obstructive airway disease) are assessed indirectly from forced expiratory manoeuvres, and abnormalities of compliance (in restrictive lung disease) are assessed indirectly from lung volume measurements.

Forced expiratory tests

Peak expiratory flow rate (PEFR) is frequently measured, despite its inability to distinguish between different types of ventilatory defect and its dependence on patient effort (Fig. 7c). The subject breathes out as hard and fast as possible from total lung capacity into a meter whose pointer records the maximum momentary flow rate achieved during the expiration. Inexpensive versions of the peak flow meter are available and used for home monitoring. It is reduced in obstructive disease, respiratory muscle weakness and often in restrictive lung disease (secondary to reduced volume). Its main value lies in monitoring diseases, especially asthma, once the diagnosis has been made.

In contrast, plots of **volume against time (spirogram)** or **airflow against volume** during a forced expiration can help to distinguish between different types of defects. The patient is asked to inhale to total lung capacity (TLC) and breathe out as hard and fast as possible to residual volume (RV). A plot of volume against time (Fig. 20a) can be produced by continuously measuring volume, either with a spirometer or by integrating a flowmeter output. If a flowmeter is used, it is also possible to compute a flow–volume plot from the same forced expiration (Fig. 7c). Flow–volume plots show characteristic shapes with different defects (Fig. 7e), such as the 'scooped out' appearance seen in obstructive airway disease.

Forced vital capacity (FVC) and **forced expiratory volume in 't' seconds (FEV$_t$)** can be read off the volume–time plot (Fig. 20a). **FEV$_1$** is extremely reproducible and correlates well with function and prognosis. It is normal for FVC and FEV$_1$ to peak in adults in the third decade and then decline by approximately 30 mL/year (Chapter 22). Forced expiratory ratio (FER = **FEV$_1$/FVC**) is normally 0.75–0.90, but higher values may occur in healthy children. FEV$_1$/FVC helps distinguish between obstructive and restrictive ventilatory defects. Typically, in obstructive lung diseases (e.g. COPD and acute asthma), the FEV$_1$/FVC is less than 0.70. If the airway obstruction is due to asthma, FEV$_1$, FVC and FEV$_1$/FVC may all increase after the inhalation of bronchodilators. In restrictive lung disease (e.g. lung fibrosis), absolute values of FEV$_1$ and FVC are reduced, but FEV$_1$/FVC is normal or high.

Forced mid-expiratory flow (FEF$_{25-75}$) is the average forced expiratory flow rate over the middle 50% of the FVC. It may be especially affected by small airway disease, but the normal range is wide.

Maximal voluntary ventilation (MVV) is measured by asking the subject to breathe as hard and fast as possible into a spirometer for 15 seconds, with the ventilation expressed in L/min. It is very dependent on effort and not very reproducible, but it may correlate well with subjective dyspnoea.

Lung volumes

Typical values for lungs volumes are given in Fig. 3, Table 1, for an average-sized healthy young man. Lung volumes are very variable and interpretation relies on comparison of the patient's measured values with the predicted values for people of the patient's age, height and gender, from nomograms constructed from large samples of healthy individuals. Some volumes can be measured using simple spirometers and some require more sophisticated techniques. **Restrictive ventilatory defects (RVDs)** are characterized by a reduction in TLC. Lung volumes such as TLC, RV and functional residual capacity (FRC) can be measured by **helium dilution** (Fig. 20b) or by **body plethysmography** (Fig. 20c). The gas dilution method is simpler for patients, but it is sensitive to gas leaks and will underestimate TLC in the presence of extensive bullous or cystic lung disease. RVDs may be caused by parenchymal lung disease (pulmonary fibrosis, scleroderma, pulmonary oedema), chest wall disease (kyphoscoliosis, massive obesity) or weak respiratory muscles (myasthenia gravis, muscular dystrophy). RV and FRC can help distinguish between these conditions, as FRC and RV are usually reduced in lung disease; whereas FRC is usually normal in muscle weakness and RV is elevated if it also affects expiratory muscles. FVC and TLC usually decline in parallel; therefore, once a RVD has been established by measurement of TLC, the progress of the disease may be followed with FVC from spirometry.

Measurement of lung compliance (Chapter 6) and **transdiaphragmatic pressure** (P_{di}) may distinguish further between RVD due to parenchymal lung disease or muscle weakness. By using two small balloon-tipped catheters, one measuring oesophageal ($P_{pleural}$) pressure and the other gastric (P_{abd}) pressure, P_{di} ($= P_{abd} - P_{pleural}$) can be measured during a maximal inspiration or sniff from FRC. Typically, in parenchymal lung disease lung compliance is low, elastic recoil pressure high and P_{di} normal; whereas in respiratory muscle weakness lung compliance is relatively normal, elastic recoil pressure low and P_{di} low.

Diffusing capacity, D_L ($=$ transfer factor, T_L), is a measure of the ability of gas to diffuse from the alveolus into pulmonary capillary blood. As discussed in Chapter 5, $D_L CO$ is used as a surrogate for $D_L O_2$, since it is simple to measure and carbon monoxide diffuses across the lung in a fashion similar to oxygen. It often helps interpretation to normalize $D_L CO$ to the alveolar volume (V_A) by calculating the coefficient, $KCO = D_L CO/V_A$. $D_L CO$ is reduced by reduced alveolar surface area, thickened alveolar–capillary membrane, reduced capillary blood volume or anaemia. Reductions in the $D_L CO$ can be caused by a variety of parenchymal diseases (idiopathic pulmonary fibrosis, emphysema, pneumonia) or vascular diseases (pulmonary hypertension, pulmonary oedema), such that the test is sensitive but not specific. Reductions in the $D_L CO$ below 50% predicted for age, sex and height are often associated with oxygen desaturation during exercise. Severe reductions in $D_L CO$ ($<20\%$ predicted) may result in resting hypoxaemia.

Arterial blood gases ($P_a O_2$, $P_a CO_2$ and pHa) and **arterial oxygen saturation** are important tests of respiratory system function and are discussed in Chapters 23 and 43.

21 Chest imaging and bronchoscopy

Evaluation of the CXR includes all the following:

(1) Date: (2) Name:

(3) AP/PA: Is it AP (anteroposterior)
    or PA (posteroanterior)?
    (Heart size cannot be measured if AP)

(4) Is it well positioned? The trachea should be
    midway between clavicles

(5) Penetration: The disc spaces should be just
    visible through the cardiac shadows
    (underpenetrated = plethoric lungs
        overpenetrated = dark lungs)

(6) Soft tissues and breast shadows
    (mastectomy in a female)

(7) Right diaphragm 2 cm higher than left
    (raised when paralysed, flat in asthma/COPD)

(8) Check ribs for fractures, metastases

(9) Right heart border = right atrium

(10) Hilium = bronchi, arteries and veins

(11) Superior vena cava

(a) Chest radiograph interpretation

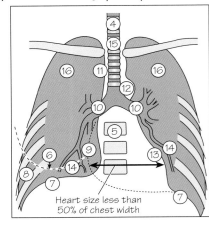

Heart size less than
50% of chest width

Normal chest X-ray

(12) Aortic arch

(13) Left heart border = left ventricle

(14) Pulmonary vessels

(15) Trachea and main bronchi

(16) Lung fields

(1) Thoracic vertebral bodies

(2) Scapula

(3) Pulmonary trunk and hilium

(4) Descending aorta

(5) Head of clavicle

(6) Trachea

(7) Arch of aorta

(8) Ascending aorta

(9) Anterior space (thymus)

(10) Heart

(11) Sternum

(12) Diaphragm

(1) Oesophagus

(2) Right lung

(3) Right main bronchus

(4) Right pulmonary artery and branches

(5) Superior vena cava

(6) Ascending aorta

(7) Pulmonary trunk

(8) Mediastinum and heart

(9) Left pulmonary artery and branches

(10) Left main bronchus

(11) Left lung

(12) Descending aorta

(b) Chest radiograph interpretation

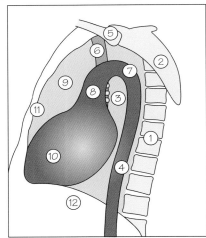

Normal lateral X-ray

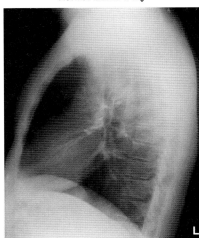

(c)

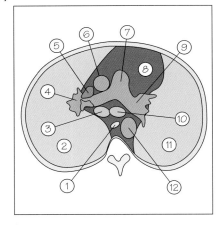

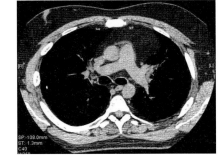

Standard (two-dimensional) chest X-rays to detect, diagnose or follow morphological abnormalities in the chest are the mainstay of thoracic radiographical imaging and account for more than 50% of procedures. Recent innovations include digital, three-dimensional computed tomography (CT) scans and physiological (positron emission tomography, ventilation–perfusion scans) imaging. Specific radiographical abnormalities are discussed in individual chapters.

Posteroanterior (PA) and lateral chest radiographs (CXRs) allow two-dimensional visualization of the lungs, great vessels, heart, diaphragm and mediastinum. PA films should be performed upright in full inspiration. Routine lateral films are not required for screening purposes. Figure 21a and 21b illustrates CXR features and interpretation. Portable anterior–posterior films (AP) in patients unable to stand magnify the heart and mediastinum and do not allow detailed visualization of lung parenchyma.

A standard PA and lateral CXR should allow visualization of both lungs, including the diaphragmatic position, as well as the normal trachea, main carina, main stem bronchi, major and minor fissures, aorta, main pulmonary arteries and heart. Understanding of the normal anatomy of a CXR is essential to allow recognition of abnormal lung parenchymal infiltrates, enlarged lymph nodes adjacent to the trachea or in the hila, enlarged pulmonary arteries, volume loss of a lobe or segment or cardiac enlargement. In the case of a suspected pleural effusion, lateral decubitus films allow visualization of as little as 50 mL of free-flowing fluid. Digital CXRs are being developed that allow more detailed views of the denser portions of the thorax and show finer detail of the lung parenchyma.

Computed tomography: a limitation of standard CXR imaging is that the two-dimensional image obscures details and averages densities in the third dimension (anterior–posterior on the PA film). CT allows thin slice axial images and fine-detailed examination of intrathoracic structures. It is more sensitive at detecting small lesions and in determining their relationship to other intrathoracic structures. Gross features are shown in Fig. 21c. Indications for CT are:
• *Bronchial carcinoma:* to detect and assess operability and prognosis of tumours (Chapter 40) by determining location, size and the presence of abnormal lymph nodes (e.g. mediastinal and axillary).
• *Lung parenchymal disease:* to detect and localize interstitial lung infiltrates, bronchiectasis, cavities, bulla, fluid collections and airway abnormalities.
• *Mediastinal masses:* to determine extent, relationship to other structures.
• *Pleural disease:* to detect asbestos-related plaques, mesothelioma and to determine the cause of pleural effusions.
• *Pulmonary emboli (PE):* administration of intravenous contrast allows imaging of the pulmonary blood vessels and detection of emboli.

Examples of CT scans are shown in several chapters. Newer technology allows complete axial scanning of the thorax with a single breath-hold.

Ventilation–perfusion (V/Q) scans are mostly performed in the evaluation of pulmonary embolism (Chapter 28). Gamma cameras can visualize radiopharmaceuticals either injected into the venous blood (perfusion) or inhaled (ventilation). Thromboembolism classically causes a V/Q mismatch, with absence of perfusion in the presence of ventilation. Unfortunately, the value of V/Q scans is limited by the observation that many PEs result in indeterminate V/Q scans that show small mismatches or matched V/Q deficits. In these cases, other studies must be utilized to demonstrate thromboemboli. Contrast CT scans are increasingly used to detect PE (see above) and are being investigated as possible replacements for V/Q scanning. Quantitative V/Q scans may be used in preparation for lung resection surgery, to assess regional lung function and estimate the amount of residual lung function.

Pulmonary angiography visualizes the vasculature following injection of contrast medium (Chapter 28). It may be required in patients with suspected pulmonary emboli but equivocal V/Q scans, pulmonary hypertension and pulmonary vascular disease, including vasculitis and arteriovenous malformations. These studies are often preceded by echocardiography to visualize right ventricular function and estimate pulmonary artery pressure using Doppler imaging.

Positron emission tomography (PET) utilizes a fluorinated analogue of glucose (FDG) to give images of the lung that highlight areas of increased glucose metabolism. Malignant cells have increased glucose uptake and appear as increased densities on PET images. Recent studies have demonstrated that PET is useful in distinguishing between benign and malignant solitary pulmonary nodules and in detecting small nodal metastases that are not detected on CT scanning. For these indications, PET has a sensitivity and specificity of 80–97% with false-positive scans seen in cases of infection or granulomatous inflammation. Whole body PET was recently used to detect clinically inapparent distant metastases.

Bronchoscopy enables direct visualization down to the fourth and fifth divisions of the endobronchial tree. Chest physicians perform most bronchoscopies as day cases under local anaesthetic in the sedated but awake patient, using a flexible fibreoptic instrument. It has the advantages of visualization of the upper lobes and is a safe technique with a low complication rate. Saturation and heart rhythm should be monitored and supplemental oxygen should be administered during the procedure. Facilities for resuscitation should always be immediately available. Thoracic surgeons may use a rigid bronchoscope in the fully anaesthetized patient. This instrument allows larger biopsies and better suctioning, and is the method of choice when removing inhaled foreign bodies. Bronchoscopy is most frequently performed to investigate if a shadow on a chest radiograph is due to a lung cancer (Chapter 40). If an endobronchial tumour is seen, biopsies for histological analysis and washings and brush samples for cytological analysis can be taken. In addition, information regarding the operability of the tumour can be obtained. Bronchoscopy can also be used to diagnose parenchymal lung disease using the technique of transbronchial biopsy, which obtains parenchymal and bronchial tissue for histological examination. Collection of bronchoalveolar fluid (bronchoalveolar lavage, BAL) is useful in diagnosing alveolitis (raised lymphocyte count in sarcoidosis), infection in the immunocompromised patient (e.g. *Pneumocystis carinii* pneumonia) and tuberculosis. Bronchoscopy also aids investigation of collapsed segments or lobes. Therapeutically, bronchoscopy is used to remove inhaled foreign bodies, to aspirate sputum plugs and secretions, to relieve stenosis by placement of stents and during treatment of endobronchial tumours with laser or endobronchial radiotherapy. Haemorrhage, pneumothorax and cardiac arrhythmia, although uncommon, are the main complications of fibreoptic bronchoscopy.

22 Public health and smoking

(a) All UK deaths in 2004

All UK deaths in 2004	587808	
Ischaemic heart disease	106081	
Non-respiratory cancer	122512	
All deaths from respiratory disease	117456	

Respiratory disease	Cases	%
• Pneumonia and TB	35814	30.5
• Lung cancer	34721	29.6
• Progressive non-malignant causes	35979	30.6
COPD + asthma	28859	24.6
Pulmonary circulatory disease	3926	3.3
Pneumoconiosis	3024	2.6
Cystic fibrosis	139	0.1
Sarcoidosis	31	0.03
• Others (congenital etc.)	10527	9

(c) Total UK emergency medical admissions by diagnosis (2004)

COPD	111000
Angina	79000
CCF	62000
Pneumonia	57000
Gastroenteritis	54000
Diabetes + complications	18000

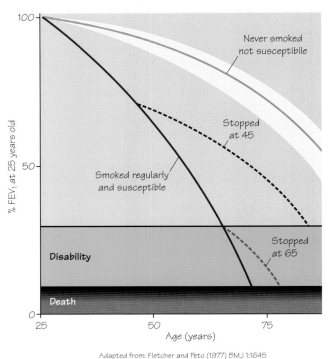

(b) Progressive decline in lung function in smokers and non-smokers and the effect of stopping smoking at 45 and 65 years old

Adapted from: Fletcher and Peto (1977) BMJ 1:1645

Respiratory disease accounts for approximately 20% of all deaths in the UK. Acute infections (30.5%), progressive non-malignant disease (30.6%) and lung cancer (29.6%) are the main causes (Fig. 22a). Annually respiratory illness is responsible for approximately 850 000 hospital admissions, 13% of emergency admissions and 10% of hospital bed days. Chest disease varies geographically in relation to socioeconomic conditions with acute infectious illness, HIV-related disease and post-tuberculous bronchiectasis more frequent in developing countries and chronic obstructive pulmonary disease (COPD), cystic fibrosis and restrictive chest wall defects (e.g. obesity hypoventilation and muscular dystrophy) more common in the USA and Europe.

Factors associated with respiratory disease

1 *Smoking-related disease (SRD)* is recognized as the single greatest cause of preventable illness and mortality. It accounts for 5 million deaths/year worldwide and 114 000 deaths/year in the UK due to a wide variety of illness including lung or non-respiratory cancers (e.g. renal and bladder), COPD, ischaemic heart disease (IHD), peripheral vascular disease, stroke, pneumonia, interstitial lung disease, venous thromboembolism, diabetes, inflammatory bowel and peptic ulcer disease. In pregnancy smoking impedes fetal growth and increases the risk of obstructive airways disease in the child. Inhaled 'second-hand'

or passive smoking increases lung cancer risk and is thought to cause approximately 12 000 deaths/year in the UK of which approximately 500 are due to workplace smoke exposure.

Tobacco smoke contains many potentially toxic gases including carbon monoxide, detected as carboxyhaemoglobin in the blood, and polycyclic aromatic hydrocarbons which cause gene mutations frequently found in primary lung cancers. Cigarette smoke accelerates normal age-related loss of lung function (Fig. 22b) and is the principal cause of COPD (Chapter 26). It also impairs epithelial ciliary function and mucociliary transport (Chapter 18), and stimulates goblet cell hyperplasia which contribute to the characteristic morning cough and excessive sputum expectoration experienced by regular smokers.

Worldwide, 20 billion cigarettes are smoked by 2 billion individuals. Oral and other smoked tobacco products are also popular. However, recent legislation, smoking bans, changes in social attitude and taxation have significantly reduced the numbers of people smoking. Consequently, in many developed countries, the incidence of SRD is no longer rising (e.g. UK), or has fallen (e.g. USA). Sadly, increased smoking in developing societies, partly due to advertising, means that the current low levels of SRD in these countries are likely to rise.

• *COPD* will rank third in worldwide burden of disease by 2020. In the UK it affects approximately 14% of people over 35 years old (7–18% of men and 3–7% of women). However, COPD is often unrecognized, despite relatively severe disease, and only 0.9 of

3 million probable UK cases have been diagnosed. In the USA approximately 2 million people have emphysema and half have reduced exercise tolerance. COPD exacerbations are the commonest cause of emergency hospital admission (Fig. 22c), with an average hospital stay of 5 days, result in 24 million lost working days annually, account for approximately 13% of adult disability and cost the economy approximately £2 billion/year in the UK.

• *Lung cancer* (Chapter 40) is the commonest cause of cancer death in men and women in the USA and Europe. Smoking increases the risk by 30-fold compared to non-smokers (<1% lifetime risk) and is dependent on dose (i.e. number of cigarettes/day, depth of inhalation, years smoked), age of onset of smoking, ethnicity (e.g. greater in blacks), geographical area (e.g. Scotland and Kentucky) and pattern of smoking (i.e. quit periods reduce future risk). Age-standardized incidence rates are approximately $65/10^5$ for males and approximately $39/10^5$ for females in the UK and USA. In Europe, Hungary has the highest ($>100/10^5$) and Sweden the lowest ($<25/10^5$) incidence. Central Africa and south central Asia have the lowest lung cancer rates. In the UK, approximately 35 000 lung cancer deaths occur annually, and after prostate cancer, it is the second commonest cancer in men, causing approximately 22 000 new cases/year and third commonest in women after breast and bowel cancer, causing approximately 16 000 new cases/year.

2 *Environmental and social factors*. Air pollution (±passive smoking), living conditions and poor sanitation increase susceptibility to acute infective diseases, asthma and hypersensitivity pneumonitis. Clean air initiatives, environmental legislation and socioeconomic programmes including better nutrition, access to clean water and education programmes (e.g. breast feeding and safe sex) have been beneficial.

• *Asthma* (Chapter 24) is the commonest respiratory disease in the UK, affecting 10–15% of the population, but there is considerable variation in worldwide prevalence, with highest levels in English-speaking countries. The cause of the recent increase in asthma incidence is unknown. Potential factors include dietary changes, improved standards of living, aeroallergens, environmental pollution, childhood infection and immunizations.

3 *Working conditions*. Protection against inhalation of mineral and organic dusts, chemicals and drugs have reduced susceptibility to occupational lung disease (e.g. coal workers' pneumoconiosis), work-related asthma and hypersensitivity pneumonitis (see Chapter 33).

Smoking cessation

In the UK, 24% of men and 23% of women smoke. However, smoking prevalence is highest in young adults (32% in 20–24 years old), manual occupations, socioeconomically deprived people and men of South Asian descent. Chinese and Indian women are least likely to smoke. Most smokers (>80%) start as teenagers and by 15 years of age 24% of girls and 16% of boys are regular smokers (average 42 cigarettes/week), despite it being illegal to sell tobacco to children. Factors associated with childhood smoking include parental smokers, one-parent families, poor academic progress and tobacco advertising.

Over two-thirds of smokers want to stop smoking. A third try every year. Successful smoking cessation reduces the risk of lung cancer by approximately 90%, but the risk is always higher than in lifelong non-smokers. The main barrier to smoking cessation is nicotine, which is highly addictive. Inhaled nicotine reaches the brain within 7–10 seconds of smoking a cigarette. It acts on brain nicotinic acetylcholine receptors (nAchR), which release neurotransmitters including nora-

drenaline (arousal, appetite reduction), serotonin (mood regulation), vasopressin (memory improvement), β-endorphin (anxiety reduction), and most importantly dopamine from the mesolimbic dopamine system or 'brain reward pathway' which elicits pleasure and is associated with the development of addictive behaviour. Smoking cessation results in physical and psychological withdrawal from the effects of these neurotransmitters and is associated with increased appetite and an average weight gain of 2 kg.

Management

Success of smoking cessation depends on both behavioural and pharmacological therapies. It is vital that the smoker is motivated to stop at the outset. To achieve sustained abstinence, the initial short-term nicotine craving is relieved with pharmacotherapy for 6–12 weeks, followed by ongoing intensive behaviour support.

a *Behavioural Strategies*

All health professionals should address smoking cessation at every opportunity. Simple clinician counselling stimulates a quit attempt in 40% of smokers. Counselling includes the 5As:

• **A**sk how much a person smokes (document pack years)
• **A**ssess risk of continued smoking and inform the patient
• **A**dvise how to stop smoking and what help is available
• **A**ssist with behavioural support or replacement therapy
• **A**rrange follow-up

Although brief counselling alone is only associated with quit rates of 1–3%, more intensive individual and group-counselling sessions with a 'quit date' can achieve abstinence in 20% at 1-year follow-up. Telephone follow-up, web-based support and multiple interviews – all improve cessation rates. Evidence for benefit with hypnosis or acupuncture is weak, but these are helpful after previous failed attempts.

b *Pharmacotherapy*

• **Nicotine replacement therapy (NRT)** ameliorates nicotine withdrawal symptoms including insomnia, irritability, anger, anxiety, poor concentration and increased appetite. It is safe, even in patients with known cardiovascular diseases. Intensive behavioural support, combined with NRT, can achieve 1-year abstinence rates of 25% (compared to ~10% with usual care). Nicotine is available as transdermal patches, gum, sublingual tablets, nasal sprays and inhalers; all are equally effective. A patch raises baseline blood nicotine levels, but combined use of a second NRT (e.g. gums, lozenges, inhalers) to provide 'bursts of nicotine' helps overcome breakthrough urges, improving long-term success.

• **Antidepressants** correct the low dopamine levels due to nicotine dependence. Smokers who are not depressed may also benefit from this approach. **Bupropion (Zyban)**, a dopamine uptake inhibitor, doubles normal quit rates. Combination with nicotine patches is not always beneficial. Bupropion is contraindicated in epilepsy and pregnancy. **Nortryptiline**, a tricyclic antidepressant, is an effective second-line agent.

• **Varenicline**, a partial agonist of nAchR, reduces withdrawal cravings and decreases the reward effects of smoking. Twelve-week quit rates comparing vareniciline, bupropion and placebo were 45, 30 and 18%, respectively, and at 12 months were 23, 16, and 9%, respectively. Varenicline is particularly effective when combined with intensive behavioural therapy.

23 Respiratory failure

(a) Causes of respiratory failure

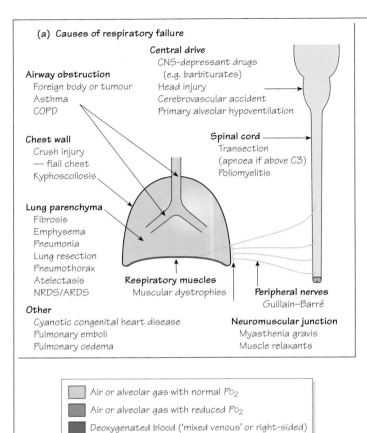

Central drive
CNS-depressant drugs
(e.g. barbiturates)
Head injury
Cerebrovascular accident
Primary alveolar hypoventilation

Airway obstruction
Foreign body or tumour
Asthma
COPD

Chest wall
Crush injury
— flail chest
Kyphoscoliosis

Spinal cord
Transection
(apnoea if above C3)
Poliomyelitis

Lung parenchyma
Fibrosis
Emphysema
Pneumonia
Lung resection
Pneumothorax
Atelectasis
NRDS/ARDS

Respiratory muscles
Muscular dystrophies

Peripheral nerves
Guillain–Barré

Other
Cyanotic congenital heart disease
Pulmonary emboli
Pulmonary oedema

Neuromuscular junction
Myasthenia gravis
Muscle relaxants

- Air or alveolar gas with normal P_{O_2}
- Air or alveolar gas with reduced P_{O_2}
- Deoxygenated blood ('mixed venous' or right-sided)
- Normal, fully oxygenated
- Incompletely oxygenated blood

(b) Mechanisms of arterial hypoxia (low P_aO_2)

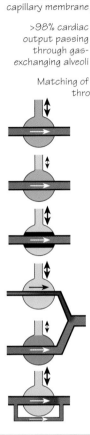

Normal
Normal alveolar-capillary membrane
>98% cardiac output passing through gas-exchanging alveoli

Normal P_{IO_2}
Normal alveolar ventilation
Normal P_aO_2

Matching of ventilation and perfusion throughout the lungs

1. **Low inspired P_{O_2}** – e.g. altitude (low P_B) or low inspired O_2 concentration → low alveolar P_{O_2}

2. **Hypoventilation** – Inadequate alveolar ventilation → low alveolar P_{O_2}

3. **Diffusion impairment** – Pulmonary capillary blood fails to reach equilibrium with alveolar gas → low pulmonary end-capillary P_{O_2}

4. **Ventilation–perfusion mismatching** – Blood from areas with high $\dot{V}_A/\dot{Q}$ mixes with blood from low $\dot{V}_A/\dot{Q}$ areas → low pulmonary venous P_{O_2}

5. **Right-to-left shunt** – Shunted blood fails to undergo gas exchanges, mixes with pulmonary capillary blood → low pulmonary venous/left ventricular P_{O_2}

(c) Effects of hypoxia and hypercapnia

	Acute	Chronic—compensation and complications
Low P_aO_2 (hypoxaemia/ hypoxia)	**Impaired CNS function:** irritability, confusion, drowsiness, convulsions, coma, death **Central cyanosis** (not very sensitive; may be absent in anaemia) **Cardiac arrhythmias** **Hypoxic vasoconstriction*** of pulmonary vessels	**Erythropoietin** from hypoxic kidney → **polycythaemia** → ↑oxygen carriage despite low P_aO_2 but if excessive (haematocrit >55%) the ↑viscosity impairs tissue blood flow **Polycythaemia** → florid complexion; increased cyanosis **Pulmonary hypertension*** → right ventricular hypertrophy **Fluid retention/right heart failure (cor pulmonale*)** → peripheral oedema/ascites/ ↑jugular venous pressure/enlarged liver
High P_aCO_2 (hypercapnia)	**Low arterial pH** (respiratory acidosis) **Peripheral vasodilatation** → warm flushed skin, bounding pulse **Cerebral vasodilatation** → ↑ intracranial pressure → headache, worse on waking if nocturnal ventilation↓ **Impaired CNS/muscle function:** irritability, confusion, somnolence, coma, tremor, myolonic jerks, hand flap **Cardiac arrhythmias**	**Renal compensation** (compensatory metabolic alkalosis) → ↑arterial [HCO_3^-] → arterial pH returned to near normal **Cerebrospinal fluid (CSF) compensation** → ↑CSF [HCO_3^-] → CSF pH returned to near normal → respiratory drive less at any given P_aCO_2 than in acute hypercapnia *Hypercapnia accentuates the effects of hypoxia on pulmonary blood vessels and therefore contributes to the development of cor pulmonale (see above)

 The Respiratory System at a Glance, 3e. By J.P.T. Ward, J. Ward, R.M. Leach. Published 2010 Blackwell Publishing Ltd.

Respiratory failure is usually said to exist when arterial P_{O_2} falls below 8 kPa (60 mmHg) when breathing air at sea level. In **type 1 respiratory failure**, the arterial hypoxia is accompanied by a normal or low arterial P_{CO_2}, whereas in **type 2 or ventilatory failure**, arterial P_{CO_2} is increased above 6.7 kPa (50 mmHg). Respiratory failure may be **acute** or **chronic**. In chronic respiratory failure, there are permanent abnormalities in blood gases, which typically worsen periodically (**acute on chronic**). This strict definition excludes some patients whose respiratory systems might otherwise be considered failing. Some patients have disabling **dyspnoea** (breathlessness) of respiratory origin but maintain P_{O_2} more than 8 kPa.

Some of the many causes of respiratory failure are listed in Fig. 23a. Symptoms and signs clearly depend on the underlying cause. Dyspnoea and **tachypnoea** (increased respiratory rate) will be prominent in severe asthma but absent in conditions with reduced central drive.

Mechanisms leading to hypoxia and hypercapnia

Of the five causes of hypoxaemia (Fig. 23b), only **hypoventilation** inevitably causes increased P_aCO_2.

$$P_aCO_2 \propto \frac{\dot{V}_{CO_2}}{\dot{V}_A} \text{ (Chapter 9)}$$

If hypoxia is out of proportion to the hypercapnia and the **A–a P_{O_2} gradient** (Chapters 14) is increased, one of the other mechanisms (3–5 in Fig. 23b) must also be present. The primary effect of **right-to-left shunts** and **ventilation–perfusion mismatching** is to raise arterial CO_2 content, but this is usually corrected or overcorrected by a reflex increase in ventilation (Chapters 13 and 14).

Thickening of the alveolar–capillary membrane in lung fibrosis may give rise to **diffusion impairment**, preventing equilibration of pulmonary capillary blood with alveolar gas, especially in exercise, when time in the capillary is reduced. However, in many conditions thought to cause diffusion impairment, there is also substantial V_A/Q mismatching, and this is probably the main cause of the hypoxia.

Effects of hypoxia and hypercapnia

The direct effects of hypoxia and hypercapnia, together with the compensations and complications that occur in chronic respiratory failure, are shown in Fig. 23c.

Although hypoxia usually offers the greatest threat to vital organs, hypercapnia and especially acidosis are also important and they often accentuate the adverse effects of each other. Hypoxia and hypercapnia are better tolerated when they develop slowly in chronic respiratory failure because of adaptations such as polycythaemia and compensatory metabolic alkalosis.

Cyanosis is a greyish-blue tinge seen when the microcirculation of a tissue contains a high concentration of deoxygenated haemoglobin. It may occur with impaired blood flow, for example in the hands and feet in circulatory shock, when it is known as **peripheral cyanosis**. When the arterial blood contains more than about 1.5–2 g/dL of deoxygenated haemoglobin, the concentration in the microcirculation reaches the critical level for cyanosis to be observable even in well-perfused tissues. This occurs with an arterial saturation of about 85% if haemoglobin concentration is normal (15 g/dL) and the resulting **central cyanosis** is

visible in the tongue and mucous membranes of the mouth. It appears at higher oxygen saturations in polycythaemic patients, whereas in severe anaemia central cyanosis may be impossible, as it would require an O_2 saturation incompatible with life.

Respiratory failure in asthma

Hypoxia in a severe asthma attack is primarily due to V_A/Q mismatching. P_aCO_2 usually falls as the attack worsens, because peripheral chemoreceptor and pulmonary receptor stimulation produce a reflex increase in ventilation despite the increased work of breathing. A raised or even apparently normal P_aCO_2 (e.g. 5.3 kPa, 40 mmHg) in a severe hypoxic asthma attack is a cause for concern, as it may indicate the onset of exhaustion and potentially life-threatening asthma.

Respiratory failure in chronic obstructive pulmonary disease

The clinical picture of severe chronic obstructive pulmonary disease (COPD) is variable (Chapter 26), but two extreme patterns – the **pink puffer** (dyspnoea, no cyanosis at rest) and the **blue bloater** (cyanosis at rest, cor pulmonale, oedema) – are recognized. The blue bloater is associated with type 2 respiratory failure. He or she has a chronically low P_aO_2 and high P_aCO_2, and these worsen with acute infections, which precipitate acute on chronic respiratory failure. Patients with chronic hypercapnia typically have a near-normal arterial pH owing to an efficient compensatory metabolic alkalosis via renal generation and retention of bicarbonate. During an acute exacerbation, P_aCO_2 may increase further and pH then falls significantly, as renal adjustments are slow. Arterial pH can therefore indicate the proportions of acute and chronic hypercapnia. Patients with chronic hypercapnia are at risk of respiratory depression and a further, potentially fatal, increase in P_aCO_2 if given high inspired oxygen (Chapter 43). This may be due to loss of hypoxic drive in the presence of reduced CO_2 sensitivity, but other mechanisms may contribute to the rise in P_aCO_2, including increased V_A/Q mismatching by the removal of hypoxic vasoconstriction. As these patients are on the steep part of the oxyhaemoglobin dissociation curve, significant improvements in arterial oxygen content can usually be achieved by small increases in F_IO_2 (to 24 or 28%). The resulting small improvement in P_aO_2 does not cause respiratory depression (Chapter 12).

Management

All patients suspected of having respiratory failure will need arterial blood gas measurement, as the severity is difficult to assess clinically. A chest X-ray helps detect possible causes and aggravating factors such as pneumonia or pneumothorax. Other investigations, including lung function tests, will depend on the clinical situation and likely underlying disease. Management will include airway maintenance, clearance of secretions, oxygen therapy (Chapter 43) and in some cases mechanical ventilation (Chapter 42). Specific therapies, such as bronchodilators and antibiotics, are directed at the underlying cause or aggravating factors. Abnormalities in haemoglobin concentration, fluid balance and cardiac output should be treated to improve tissue oxygen delivery and increase mixed venous oxygen content, which in turn will also reduce the effects of venous admixture on arterial oxygenation.

24 Asthma: pathophysiology

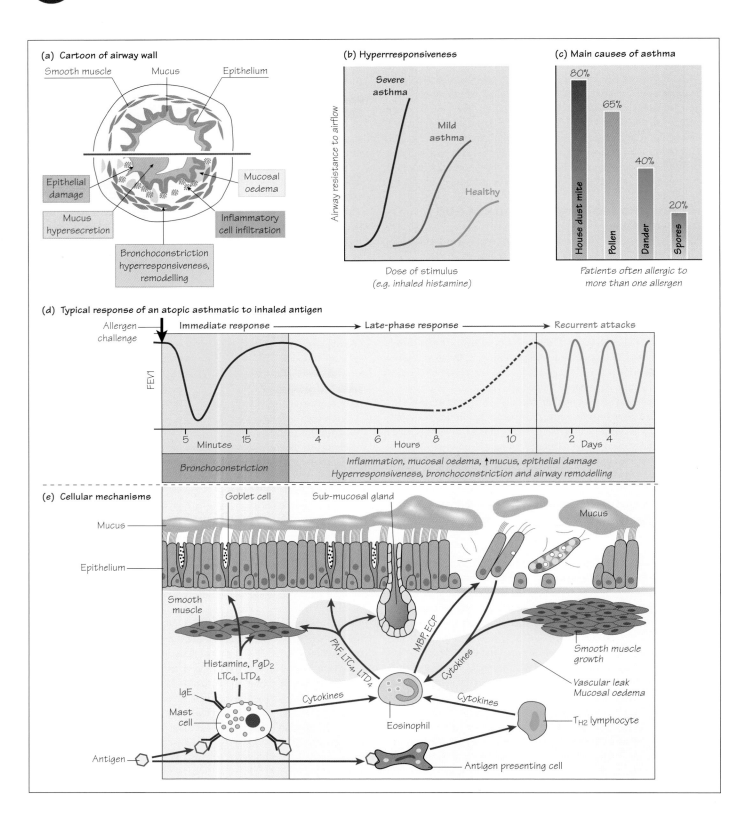

(a) Cartoon of airway wall

Smooth muscle • Mucus • Epithelium

Epithelial damage
Mucus hypersecretion
Bronchoconstriction hyperresponsiveness, remodelling
Mucosal oedema
Inflammatory cell infiltration

(b) Hyperrresponsiveness

Severe asthma
Mild asthma
Healthy

Airway resistance to airflow

Dose of stimulus (e.g. inhaled histamine)

(c) Main causes of asthma

80% House dust mite
65% Pollen
40% Dander
20% Spores

Patients often allergic to more than one allergen

(d) Typical response of an atopic asthmatic to inhaled antigen

Allergen challenge
Immediate response — Late-phase response — Recurrent attacks

FEV1

5 Minutes 15   4   6 Hours 8   10   2 Days 4

Bronchoconstriction | Inflammation, mucosal oedema, ↑mucus, epithelial damage Hyperresponsiveness, bronchoconstriction and airway remodelling

(e) Cellular mechanisms

Mucus • Goblet cell • Sub-mucosal gland • Mucus
Epithelium
Smooth muscle
Histamine, PgD$_2$ LTC$_4$, LTD$_4$
IgE
Mast cell
Antigen
PAF, LTC$_4$, LTD$_4$
MBP, ECP
Cytokines
Cytokines
Cytokines
Cytokines
Eosinophil
Smooth muscle growth
Vascular leak Mucosal oedema
T$_{H2}$ lymphocyte
Antigen presenting cell

 The Respiratory System at a Glance, 3e. By J.P.T. Ward, J. Ward, R.M. Leach. Published 2010 Blackwell Publishing Ltd.

Asthma is an inflammatory disorder of the airways. Patients suffer from episodes of cough, wheezing, chest tightness and/or dyspnoea (breathlessness), which are often worse at night or early in the morning. Asthma can be usefully defined as 'a chronic inflammatory disorder characterized by increased responsiveness of the bronchi to various innocuous stimuli, manifested by widespread and variable airway narrowing that varies in severity either spontaneously or with treatment'. The major characteristics of asthma are (Fig. 24a):

1 Narrowing of the airways and impeded airflow, commonly reversible spontaneously or following treatment.

2 Non-specific airway **hyperresponsiveness** to a range of normally innocuous stimuli (e.g. cold air, irritants and pollutants) and airway spasmogens leading to bronchoconstriction (Fig. 24b).

3 Increased mucosal inflammation and recruitment of **inflammatory cells** (eosinophils, mast cells, neutrophils, T lymphocytes) to the airways.

There is also **hypersecretion of mucus**, which can lead to blockage of airways with **mucus plugs**, and swelling of mucosa due to inflammation-associated vascular leak and consequent **oedema** of the airway wall, all of which further limit airflow. Damage to the epithelium (**epithelial shedding**) is reflected by whorls of epithelial cells (Curschmann's spirals) in the mucus, which also contains eosinophil cell membranes (Charcot–Leyden crystals). In chronic asthma **remodelling of the airway wall** structure occurs, including increased bronchial smooth muscle content. This causes irreversible narrowing of the airways and limits the effectiveness of bronchodilators.

Prevalence

Asthma is increasing in prevalence, particularly in the Western world, where more than 5% of the population may be symptomatic and receiving treatment. There has been a concomitant increase in mortality, despite improved treatment. In the UK, one in seven of the population has allergic disease and over 9 million people will have wheezed in the last year. The number of teenagers with asthma has nearly doubled over the last 12 years. Asthma is least common in the Far East and most common in the UK, Australia and New Zealand. There is some correlation with Westernized lifestyles, including living conditions that favour house dust mites and atmospheric pollution. Many factors can precipitate an asthma attack or worsen symptoms, including exposure to specific **antigens**, **tobacco smoke** and **exhaust fumes**, and **emotional stress**. Exercise (**exercised-induced asthma**) and inhalation of cold air often precipitate wheezing in asthmatics, probably via drying and cooling of the bronchial epithelium, and is common in children. Certain **viral infections** (rhinovirus, parainfluenza, respiratory syncytial virus) are associated with asthma attacks. There may also be a genetic component to asthma. Importantly, 20% of the working population may be susceptible to **occupational asthma** due to their working environment (Chapter 33).

Classification

Asthma can be classified as **extrinsic**, having a definite external cause, and **intrinsic**, where no external cause can be identified. Extrinsic asthma commonly occurs as a result of an allergic response, with development of **IgE antibodies** to specific antigens (**allergic** or **atopic asthma**) and tends to start in childhood with symptoms becoming less severe with age; approximately 80% of asthmatics are atopic. Intrinsic asthma generally appears in adults and is **IgE-independent**.

Atopic asthma

Individuals who readily produce IgE to common antigens are prone to allergic asthma. Major antigens include proteins in fecal pellets from **house dust mite** (*Dermatophagoids pteronyssinus*; **DerP**) – the most common cause of asthma worldwide – grass and tree **pollen**, dander (skin flakes) from **domestic pets** and **fungal spores** (Fig. 24c). Genetic factors, atmospheric pollution and maternal smoking in pregnancy all predispose to raised IgE levels and later development of asthma and airway hyperresponsiveness.

Inhalation of allergens by atopic individuals initiates an **immediate response** (bronchoconstriction) that usually subsides within 2 hours (Fig. 24d); this is reversible with bronchodilators such as β_2-adrenoceptor agonists (Chapter 25). This is often followed 3–12 hours later by a **late-phase response** with bronchoconstriction, airway inflammation and oedema, and hyperresponsiveness (Fig. 24d), which is less susceptible to bronchodilators. Some materials (e.g. **isocyanates**) cause only an **isolated late phase**. The increased hyperresponsiveness may promote **recurrent asthma attacks** over several days.

The immediate response is an example of **type I hypersensitivity**. It is caused by antigen/IgE-induced **mast cell degranulation** and release of **histamine**, **prostaglandin D$_2$** (PgD_2) and **leukotriene C$_4$** and **D$_4$** (LTC_4, LTD_4); these cause bronchoconstriction, increased mucus production and vascular leak (Fig. 24e). The late phase (an example of **type IV** or **cell-based hypersensitivity**) is primarily due to inflammation. Mast cells and, in particular, activated **T$_{H2}$ lymphocytes** release **cytokines** (cellular mediators) that attract **eosinophils** and **neutrophils** to the area. T$_{H2}$ lymphocytes are a specific type of T$_H$ cell that are also activated by **antigen presenting cells** (see Chapter 18), but unlike T$_{H1}$ cells release cytokines such as IL-5 which recruit eosinophils. Asthma is therefore sometimes described as a T$_{H2}$-driven disease, and may involve an imbalance between T$_{H1}$ and T$_{H2}$ lymphocytes.

Consequently, eosinophils are present in large numbers in asthmatic bronchi, and release **leukotrienes**, platelet-activating factor (**PAF**), **major basic protein** (MBP) and **eosinophil cationic protein** (ECP). MBP and ECP contribute to epithelial cell damage, causing increased permeability to allergens, release of cytokines that attract more eosinophils (Fig. 24e), and exposure of C-fibre sensory nerve endings which release proinflammatory tachykinins. Asthmatic smooth muscle also produces cytokines. Important cytokines involved in asthma include IL-5, IL-13, eotaxin, RANTES and granulocyte macrophage colony-stimulating factor (GM-CSF).

Drug-associated asthma

Aspirin and other non-steroidal anti-inflammatory drugs (NSAIDs) promote asthmatic attacks in 5% of asthmatics. They inhibit the cyclooxygenase (COX) pathway that synthesizes prostaglandins and shift arachidonic acid metabolism from COX towards the lipoxygenase pathway and production of LTC_4 and LTD_4. Aspirin-induced asthma is partially reversed by antileukotriene therapy (Chapter 25).

The bronchi have little sympathetic innervation, but circulating epinephrine (adrenaline) acting via β_2-adrenoceptors on smooth muscle causes bronchodilatation. Consequently β-adrenoceptor antagonists can cause bronchoconstriction in asthmatics. This may even occur with nominally β_1-selective drugs, and their use for cardiovascular disease should be avoided in asthmatics.

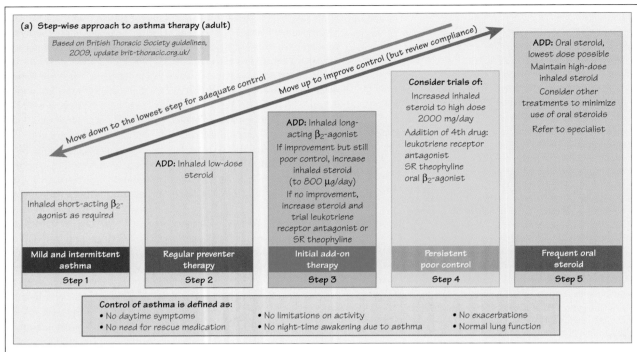

(a) Step-wise approach to asthma therapy (adult)

Based on British Thoracic Society guidelines, 2009, update brit-thoracic.org.uk/

Move down to the lowest step for adequate control

Move up to improve control (but review compliance)

Inhaled short-acting β₂-agonist as required

| Mild and intermittent asthma | | Regular preventer therapy | | Initial add-on therapy | | Persistent poor control | | Frequent oral steroid | |

ADD: Inhaled low-dose steroid

ADD: Inhaled long-acting β₂-agonist
If improvement but still poor control, increase inhaled steroid (to 800 µg/day)
If no improvement, increase steroid and trial leukotriene receptor antagonist or SR theophyline

Consider trials of:
Increased inhaled steroid to high dose 2000 mg/day
Addition of 4th drug: leukotriene receptor antagonist
SR theophyline
oral β₂-agonist

ADD: Oral steroid, lowest dose possible
Maintain high-dose inhaled steroid
Consider other treatments to minimize use of oral steroids
Refer to specialist

Mild and intermittent asthma	Regular preventer therapy	Initial add-on therapy	Persistent poor control	Frequent oral steroid
Step 1	Step 2	Step 3	Step 4	Step 5

Control of asthma is defined as:
- No daytime symptoms
- No need for rescue medication
- No limitations on activity
- No night-time awakening due to asthma
- No exacerbations
- Normal lung function

(b) Most common drug classes used in asthma

Type	Route and example	Effect	Adverse effects
β₂–agonist (adrenoreceptor agonists)	Inhaled, oral, intravenous (IV) Short-acting: salbutamol (albuterol) Long-acting: salmeterol, formoterol	Bronchodilators May stabilize mast cells (increase cAMP)	Muscle tremor (most common) Tachycardia, palpitations (high dose)
Corticosteroids	Inhaled: Beclometasone proprionate Oral: Prednisolene IV: Hydrocortisone	Anti-inflammatory (Suppress activation of inflammatory genes)	Inhaled: oral candidiasis, cough, hoarseness Oral/high dose: Retarded growth, water retention, osteoporosis, hypertension, weight gain, eye problems, diabetes, psychosis
Xanthines	Oral, IV: Theophylline, aminophylline Slow release (SR) formulations	Bronchodilators Some anti-inflammatory action (increase cAMP)	Headache, nausea, diuresis, cardiac arrhythmias, vomiting, epilepsy; many drug interactions affect xanthine plasma levels
Muscarinic receptor antagonists	Inhaled: Ipratropium bromide	Bronchodilators Reduce mucus secretion (block cholinergic effects)	Rare, bitter taste
Antileukotrienes Receptor antagonist Lipoxygenase inhibitor	Oral: Montelukast, zafirlukast Zileuton (not licensed in UK)	Bronchodilators May reduce mucosal oedema (block action of LTC₄, LTD₄)	None-significant described

(c) Pressurized metered dose inhaler

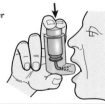

- Remove the cap and shake the inhaler
- Tilt the head back slightly and exhale
- Position the inhaler in the mouth (or preferably just in front of the open mouth)
- During a slow inspiration, press down the inhaler to release the medication
- Continue inhalation to full inspiration
- Hold breath for 10 seconds
- Actuate only one puff per inhalation

The Respiratory System at a Glance, 3e. By J.P.T. Ward, J. Ward, R.M. Leach. Published 2010 Blackwell Publishing Ltd.

Management of asthma should encompass assessment of severity and efficacy of therapy, identification and removal of precipitating factors, therapy to reverse bronchoconstriction and inflammation, patient and family participation and education. Diagnosis is determined on the basis of a characteristic pattern of signs and symptoms in the absence of alternative explanations.

Assessment

Lung function: Primary assessment is with spirometry. Asthma is probable when inhaled bronchodilators cause more than 15% improvement in forced expiratory volume in 1 second (FEV_1) or peak expiratory flow rate (PEFR) (Chapter 20). The absence of improvement does not rule out asthma – the patient could be in remission and chronic severe asthma is poorly reversible. Airway resistance is least at midday and greatest at 3–4 a.m. Serial measurements of PEFR in the morning, midday and on retiring are useful for identifying the enhanced variation in airflow limitation characteristic of asthma and for assessing response to therapy over time. Poorly controlled asthma shows a characteristic morning fall in PEFR (**morning dipping**). Occupational asthma is suggested when PEFR improves after a break from work. Lung function tests are often coupled with exercise tests in children, who often exhibit exercise-induced asthma.

Bronchial provocation tests can determine **hyperresponsiveness** (Chapter 24) when asthma is suspected but spirometry is not diagnostic. Patients inhale increasing doses of histamine or methacholine (acetylcholine analogue) until FEV_1 declines by 20%. The dose at which this occurs ($PD_{20}FEV_1$) is greatly reduced in asthmatics, who are always hyperresponsive (Fig. 24b).

Skin prick tests identify extrinsic factors. Development of a wheal around the prick site indicates allergen sensitivity. Exposure to identified allergens should be minimized (e.g. replacement of furnishings to reduce house dust mite, removal of pets). Only 50% of patients with occupational asthma are cured by avoidance of precipitating factors.

Therapy

The goal is long-term control, and all patients except those with the mildest symptoms should receive anti-inflammatory drugs as well as bronchodilators. International guidelines favour **step-wise treatment regimens** (Fig. 25a). Asthma therapy is centred on **inhaled** compounds (Fig. 25b), which maximize bronchial delivery while minimizing systemic side effects. Metered dose inhalers (**MDI**) are the commonest delivery system, although only approximately 15–20% of the dose may reach the lungs (Fig. 25c); this can be improved by use of spacers. Asthma drugs are often called **relievers**, bronchodilators that relieve acute symptoms, or **preventers**, prophylactic and anti-inflammatory drugs that relieve chronic symptoms and hyperresponsiveness; some have both properties. Histamine antagonists have not proved useful in asthma.

Short-acting β_2-adrenoceptor agonists (e.g. salbutamol) are rapid and powerful bronchodilators and are of first choice for alleviating acute symptoms. They activate adenylate cyclase to increase cyclic adenosine monophosphate (cAMP). In addition to bronchodilation, they also reduce activation of mast cells. **Long-acting β_2-agonists** (e.g. salmeterol) are used prophylactically, but must only be used for patients already on steroids (see below). Long-term use of β_2-agonists is associated with reduced effectiveness (**tolerance**).

Corticosteroids (e.g. beclometasone) are the most important anti-inflammatory (preventer) drugs, and suppress inflammatory gene activation. Steroids reduce eosinophil numbers and activity of macrophages and lymphocytes. **Inhaled steroids** are the mainstay of long-term asthma therapy. However, they can have significant side effects, including oral candidiasis (5%) and hoarseness. Growth may be retarded in children receiving high-dose inhaled corticosteroids. **Oral corticosteroids** such as prednisolone may be required in patients whose asthma cannot be controlled by inhaled steroids, but the danger of adverse effects is much greater. **Combination therapies** containing both steroid and long-acting β_2-agonists are commonly used for moderate/severe asthmatics.

Muscarinic receptor antagonists (e.g. ipratropium) block the effects of acetylcholine from parasympathetic nerves to smooth muscle and mucus glands. They are moderately effective bronchodilators and reduce mucus secretion. They are slower and less effective than β_2-agonists, and more useful against irritant than allergen-induced responses.

Xanthines such as theophylline have bronchodilatory and some anti-inflammatory actions and are taken orally. They inhibit phosphodiesterases that break down cAMP. Limitations include numerous side effects and a narrow therapeutic range; these are partially overcome by slow-release (SR) preparations. Xanthines are used as second-line drugs in asthma, particularly when β_2-agonists are ineffective at controlling symptoms and in steroid-resistant asthma.

Antileukotriene therapy includes cysLT receptor (LTC_4/D_4) antagonists (e.g. montelukast) and 5-lipoxygenase inhibitors (e.g. zileuton). Both have equal efficacy for bronchoconstriction caused by allergens, exercise and cold air. They are effective in aspirin-sensitive asthma, indicating the key role leukotrienes have in this condition (Chapter 24). Antileukotrienes improve lung function in mild and moderate asthmatics, but the greatest benefit may be for severe asthmatics taking steroids. Both drug types are taken orally and are relatively long-lasting, with few adverse effects.

Cromones (sodium cromoglicate, nedocromil) inhibit activation of mast cells and eosinophils, and may suppress sensory nerves and release of neuropeptides (Chapter 24). They are only effective prophylactically. Use has declined as they are less effective and more expensive than modern low-dose steroids, but are useful when steroids cannot be used.

Allergen-specific immunotherapy: Recombinant anti-IgE antibody (omalizumab) has been shown to be effective in moderate to severe allergic asthma, by reducing levels of antigen-specific IgE. Promising results have been obtained in trials of anti-cytokine antibodies (e.g. anti-IL-13, anti-IL-5). Both require specialist treatment centres.

Bronchial thermoplasty uses heat to reduce smooth muscle mass and function in medium airways, and has been used successfully in severe uncontrolled asthmatics.

Poorly controlled asthma is often related to poor compliance with treatment regimens – for example, due to peer pressure in children. Poor inhaler techniques are common. Compliance may also be poor when asthma is apparently controlled, so patients stop preventer therapies (e.g. steroids) because they are 'cured'. Patient education and training are therefore key to asthma therapy.

Severe uncontrolled asthma

Requires immediate treatment and hospitalization. **Indications:** inability to complete sentences ('telegraph speaking'), high respiratory rate, tachycardia, PEFR less than 50% predicted. Becomes **life-threatening** with one or more of: PEFR less than 33% predicted, hypoxaemia, hypercapnia, silent chest, exhaustion. **Treatment:** immediate nebulized β_2-agonists $+/-$ ipratropium delivered in oxygen and intravenous steroids, with subsequent oral steroids. In unresolving cases, intravenous β_2-agonists or xanthines and ventilation may be required.

(a) Risk factors for COPD

Smoking
Age >50 years old; prevalence ~5–10%
Male gender
Childhood chest infections
Airways hyperreactivity
• asthma/atopy
Low socioeconomic status
α_1-Antitrypsin deficiency
Heavy metal exposure
• cadmium
Atmospheric pollution

(b) Pathophysiology of chronic bronchitis and emphysema

Chronic bronchitis

Pressure collapsing airway in expiration balanced by lung's elastic recoil and airway held open

Normal lung parenchyma provides lung's elastic recoil

Mucosal inflammation and mucous secretion cause narrowing (± obstruction) of some airways

Poor ventilation and collapse of some alveoli (e.g. mucous plugs) cause V/Q mismatch + hypoxaemia

(c) Spirometry. FEV_1/FVC ratio decreases in COPD

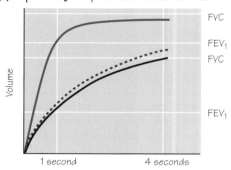

FVC
FEV_1
FVC

FEV_1

1 second   4 seconds

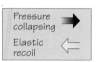

Pressure collapsing →
Elastic recoil ←

Normal ────
FEV_1/FVC = >0.8

COPD ────
FEV_1/FVC = <0.8

COPD ┄┄┄┄
Irreversible with bronchodilators
<15% increase in FEV_1

Emphysema

Pressure collapsing airway in expiration is greater than lung's elastic recoil causing distal airways collapse

Loss of alveolar septa and capillaries reduces the lung's elastic recoil. Large air spaces (bullae) develop

Increased upper airway pressure (purse-lip breathing, CPAP) will tend to hold airways open and allows increased alveolar emptying

Collapse of distal airways in expiration causes gas trapping and alveolar hyper-inflation

(d) Typical signs and symptoms of COPD

Chronic bronchitis	Emphysema
Chronic cough, producing sputum Hypoventilation, little respiratory effort Cyanosis, hypoxaemia with secondary polycythaemia CO_2 retention/chronic hypercapnia — leading to peripheral vasodilatation and bounding pulse Oedema Cor pulmonale **Normal** lung volumes, D_LCO, lung compliance	Chronic breathlessness (dyspnoea) Cyanosis unusual; normoxic at rest, hypoxic on exercise Barrel chest (hyperinflation), underweight Rarely exhibit oedema or cor pulmonale **Increased** TLC, RV, lung compliance **Reduced** D_LCO
Note: Most patients may present with both chronic bronchitis and emphysema	

Chronic obstructive pulmonary disease (COPD) is characterized by *irreversible* expiratory airflow obstruction, hyperinflation, mucus hypersecretion and increased work of breathing. COPD encompasses **chronic bronchitis** and **emphysema**, which often present together but reflect different underlying processes. Typically, smoking and other risk factors (Fig. 26a) accelerate the normal age-related decline in lung function (Chapter 22), and cause chronic respiratory symptoms interposed with intermittent **acute exacerbations**, eventually leading to disability and **respiratory failure** (Chapter 23). Chronic hypoxaemia in COPD can lead to **pulmonary hypertension** (Chapter 27). Asthma is not classified as COPD as it is *reversible* (Chapters 24 and 25).

Diagnosis and pathophysiology

COPD is diagnosed by airflow obstruction indicated by a **reduced FEV_1/FVC ratio** of less than 0.7, which is irreversible ($<15\%$ increase in FEV_1) with bronchodilator or steroid therapy (Fig. 26c; Chapter 20). Restrictive lung disease (e.g. fibrosis) should be excluded. Patients with COPD have symptoms of **dyspnoea** (breathlessness) at rest or on exertion. Many asymptomatic smokers have lung function abnormalities that predate symptoms, which may be prevented by early smoking cessation. Although chronic bronchitis and emphysema most often coexist, they reflect different underlying processes (Fig. 26b) with differing signs and symptoms (Fig. 26d).

Chronic bronchitis is associated with airways obstruction caused by **chronic mucosal inflammation**, **mucous gland hypertrophy** and **mucus hypersecretion**, coupled with **bronchospasm** (Fig. 26b). It is defined by daily morning of cough and excessive mucus production for 3 months in 2 successive years, in the absence of airway tumour, acute/chronic infection or uncontrolled cardiac disease. Most patients have normal total lung capacity (TLC), functional residual capacity (FRC), residual volume (RV), D_LCO (diffusing capacity) and static lung compliance (Chapter 20). Patients with advanced chronic bronchitis have reduced respiratory drive and CO_2 **retention**, which is associated with bounding pulse, vasodilatation, confusion, headache, flapping tremor and papilloedema. **Hypoxaemia** is mostly due to V_A/Q mismatch (Fig. 26b; Chapter 14), and leads to **polycythaemia** (increased red cells) and **increased pulmonary artery pressure** (pulmonary hypertension) due to **hypoxic pulmonary vasoconstriction**. The resulting impairment of the right side of the heart function leads to renal fluid retention, raised central venous pressure and **peripheral oedema**, subsequently leading to **cor pulmonale** (fluid retention/heart failure secondary to lung disease). Pulmonary hypertension is potentiated by extensive capillary loss in late disease. There are no radiographical signs, diagnostic of chronic bronchitis.

Emphysema is caused by progressive destruction of alveolar septa and capillaries, leading to development of **enlarged airways and airspaces** (bullae), decreased lung elastic recoil and increased airway collapsibility. Airway obstruction is caused by collapse of distal airways during expiration due to loss of elastic radial traction present in the normal lung (Fig. 26b). The resulting **hyperinflation** enhances expiratory airflow, but inspiratory muscles work at a mechanical disadvantage. The pathophysiology of emphysema may involve an imbalance between inflammatory cell proteases and antiprotease defences (Chapter 18). Centrilobular emphysema is associated with cigarette smoking and predominantly involves the upper lung zones. Panacinar emphysema is associated with α_1-**antitrypsin deficiency** (Chapter 18) and predominantly involves the lower lung zones. Patients with emphysema typically have airflow obstruction with elevated TLC, FRC and RV, reduced D_LCO and increased static lung compliance. Such patients tend to be breathless and tachypnoeic (fast respiratory rate) at rest, with signs of hyperinflation and malnutrition including **barrel chest** and thin body, use of accessory respiratory muscles and **purse-lipped breathing**. The latter increases pressure in the upper airways and thus limits distal airway collapse. Auscultation reveals distant breath sounds with a prolonged expiratory wheeze. Blood gases are normal at rest, with marked O_2 desaturation during exertion. Radiographically, emphysema may appear as hyperinflated lungs with a large retrosternal airspace and flat diaphragms. When the condition is advanced, there may be areas with a lack of vascularity or visualization of bullae. High-resolution computed tomography (CT) is useful to demonstrate enlarged airspaces and air trapping.

Management

No specific therapy reverses COPD, but treatment can slow disease progression, ease chronic symptoms and prevent acute exacerbations. Smoking cessation is critical. Pharmacological therapy has similarities to that of asthma (Chapter 25).

Inhaled β_2-**agonists** (e.g. salbutamol) and **anticholinergics** may improve symptoms and lung function, and have additive effects when combined. **Xanthines** have negligible effects on spirometry, yet may improve exercise performance and blood gases. Patients producing large amounts of sputum may benefit from **mucolytics**. **Inhaled corticosteroids** are recommended in severe disease ($FEV_1 < 50\%$ predicted). Long-term **oral corticosteroids** (to reduce inflammation) are best avoided as they improve function in less than 25% of COPD patients but cause significant side effects. **Pulmonary rehabilitation** strengthens respiratory muscles and improves quality of life and exercise tolerance while reducing hospitalizations but has no effect on lung function. O_2 **therapy** prolongs life in patients with resting daytime hypoxaemia by slowing progression of cor pulmonale. O_2 should be utilized as much as possible, as benefit increases with use. Patients with nocturnal or exercise desaturation benefit from supplemental O_2 at night or during exercise. In α_1-**antitrypsin deficiency**, replacement therapy can increase plasma and lung antiprotease levels; however, the benefits on lung function and survival are controversial. Surgical **lung volume reduction** or **transplantation** may be indicated in advanced COPD for carefully selected patients.

Prevention of acute COPD exacerbations includes pneumococcal and influenza vaccination. Patients with any combination of increased dyspnoea, increased sputum or purulent sputum benefit from antibiotics targeted against common respiratory pathogens (e.g. *Haemophilus influenzae*). Short courses of oral corticosteroids improve lung function and hasten recovery in patients with acute exacerbations.

Overall prognosis for COPD patients is dependent on the severity of airflow obstruction. Patients with a FEV_1 less than 0.8 L have a yearly mortality of approximately 25%. Patients with cor pulmonale, hypercapnia, ongoing cigarette smoking and weight loss have a worse prognosis. Death usually occurs from infection, acute respiratory failure, pulmonary embolus or cardiac arrhythmia.

27 Pulmonary hypertension

(a) Causes of pulmonary hypertension (Venice/WHO 2003)

1. **Pulmonary arterial hypertension (PAH):**
   1.1 Idiopathic (IPAH)
   1.2 Familial (FPAH) (e.g. mutation in bone morphogentic protein receptor (BMPR)
   1.3 Associated with (APAH) connective tissue diseases, congenital systemic-
       pulmonary shunts, portal hypertension (cirrhosis), HIV infection, drugs and
       toxins + disorders (e.g. thyroid)
   1.4 Associated venous or capillary involvement: pulmonary veno-occlusive disease
       and pulmonary capillary haemangiomatosis
   1.5 Persistent PH in the newborn (PPHN)
2. **PH associated with left heart disease** including left-sided valvular heart disease
3. **PH associated with lung diseases and/or hypoxia** including COPD, interstitial
   lung disease, sleep-disordered breathing, hypoventilation, high altitude exposure +
   developmental abnormalities
4. **PH due to chronic thrombotic and/or embolic disease** including thromboembolic
   obstruction of pulmonary artery and non-thrombotic pulmonary embolism
   (e.g. tumour, parasites)

Secondary to respiratory disease:
Alveolar hypoxia -
COPD (Chapter 26)
Interstitial lung disease (Chapter 30)
ARDS (Chapter 41)
Sleep-disordered breathing (Chapter 44)

Secondary to thrombotic disease:
Chronic thromboembolic disease
Embolic obliterative disease

**Disorders directly affecting
the vasculature:**
Interstitial lung disease (Chapter 30)
Vasculitis (Chapter 29)
Emphysema (Chapter 26)
Schistosomiasis

Pulmonary venous hypertension:
Left ventricular heart failure
Mitral stenosis/insufficiency
Fibrosing mediastinitis
Left atrial myxoma
Veno-occlusive disease

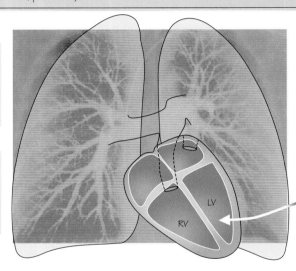

(b) Evaluation of suspected pulmonary hypertension

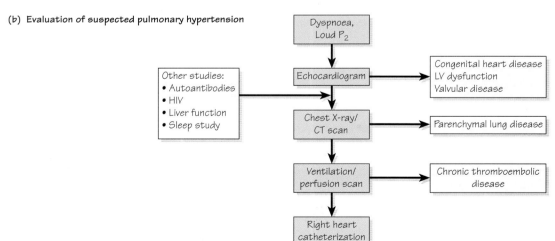

Dyspnoea, Loud P$_2$

Other studies:
• Autoantibodies
• HIV
• Liver function
• Sleep study

Echocardiogram → Congenital heart disease / LV dysfunction / Valvular disease

Chest X-ray/ CT scan → Parenchymal lung disease

Ventilation/ perfusion scan → Chronic thromboembolic disease

Right heart catheterization

 The Respiratory System at a Glance, 3e. By J.P.T. Ward, J. Ward, R.M. Leach. Published 2010 Blackwell Publishing Ltd.

Pulmonary hypertension (PH) is defined as a mean pulmonary artery (PA) pressure of more than **25 mmHg** at rest or more than **30 mmHg** during exercise (normal value ~14 mmHg mean). A rise in PA pressure can be due to increased **pulmonary vascular resistance** (e.g. hypoxia and embolism), pulmonary blood flow and **back-pressure** (pulmonary venous pressure, e.g. left heart failure). PH is most commonly caused by another disorder (**secondary PH**). More rarely it is due to a disorder of the pulmonary circulation itself, when it is termed **pulmonary arterial hypertension** (PAH). Idiopathic PAH (IPAH) has no apparent cause. The Venice (WHO) classification of PH is shown in Fig. 27a.

Types of pulmonary hypertension

Secondary to respiratory disease: most common, due to hypoxaemia which causes small pulmonary arteries to constrict (**hypoxic pulmonary vasoconstriction**). PH is often associated with COPD (Chapter 26). Any condition leading to hypoxia can cause PH, including sleep-disordered breathing (Chapter 44) and exposure to altitude (Chapter 15).

Pulmonary venous hypertension: increased left atrial (LA) pressure, most commonly due to left ventricular dysfunction as in **congestive heart failure**, leads to elevation of PA pressure by increasing back-pressure through the lungs. **Mitral insufficiency** or **stenosis** may also increase PA pressure enough to cause hypertension. In these cases, patients will often have signs of pulmonary capillary hypertension such as crackles. Echocardiography should demonstrate LA enlargement.

Secondary to thrombotic disease: acute and chronic venous **thromboembolism** causes PH by mechanical obstruction of the proximal or distal pulmonary arteries. In acute thromboembolism, a component of vasospasm is also present, as the platelet-rich thromboembolus releases vasoactive mediators such as thromboxane, serotonin or platelet-activating factor. This form is also associated with sickle cell disease.

Disorders directly affecting the vasculature: increases in pulmonary vascular resistance may occur in the veins, capillaries or arteries. Increases in **capillary resistance** are common and may occur in any lung disease that causes capillary distortion or reduction in surface area. **Interstitial lung diseases** (Chapters 30 & 31) such as pulmonary **fibrosis**, **scleroderma** or **sarcoidosis** cause capillary distortion, as lung parenchyma is affected. Destruction of capillaries occurs in **emphysema** (Chapter 26) or pneumonectomy. In schistosomiasis (bilharzia) the parasitic worms can block pulmonary capillaries.

Pulmonary arterial hypertension includes IPAH, PH associated with conditions such as collagen vascular disease, HIV and portal hypertension but where no causal relationship can be determined, and persistent pulmonary hypertension of the newborn (PPHN). IPAH is rare (1–2 per million population) and its pathogenesis is unclear. Genetic abnormalities, in particular related to bone morphogenic protein and serotonin transporters, may predispose patients to IPAH, but although some cases are clearly **familial** with autosomal dominant inheritance, other are **sporadic** with no family history. IPAH is more common in women than men (ratio 2:1) and most prevalent between 20 and 40 years of age. Certain appetite-suppressant drugs affecting serotonin (e.g. fenfluramine) are associated with a 30-fold increase in risk after 3 months. Remodelling of pulmonary arterioles is characteristic of IPAH, although in some patients a component of arterial vasospasm is suggested by the effect of vasodilators.

Clinical features

Development of PH can substantially increase morbidity and mortality. The prognosis for COPD patients with PH is much worse, with a 5-year survival for of less than 10% if PA pressure is more than 45 mmHg compared with more than 90% with PA pressure less than 25 mmHg. Mean survival without treatment in IPAH is 2 years. Patients usually die from **progressive right-sided heart failure**. Chronic PH can lead to pulmonary vascular **remodelling** and thickening of the pulmonary vasculature, reducing the efficacy of vasodilators. PH is generally slow to develop and presents with non-specific symptoms, including dyspnoea on exertion, shortness of breath, palpitations, chest pain, light-headedness and syncope. Signs are difficult to elicit early and may only include an increased pulmonic component of the second heart sound. With more severe hypertension, **right ventricular dysfunction** will be apparent, including jugular venous distension, right ventricular heave, pedal oedema and hepatic enlargement. Detection of PH requires a high index of suspicion, because signs and symptoms are non-specific and the diagnosis requires further testing; there is significant underdiagnosis.

Diagnosis

Evaluation of patients with suspected PH (Fig. 27b) begins with **echocardiography**, allowing calculation of right ventricular systolic pressure and visualization of left atrium (LA), mitral valve, right ventricle and congenital abnormalities. If PH is found in conjunction with an enlarged LA, it is most likely due to either left ventricular or mitral disease. Chest radiology, pulmonary function testing and measurement of arterial oxygen allow detection of parenchymal disease or hypoxia. In the absence of LA enlargement or pulmonary parenchymal disease, further evaluation of pulmonary arteries is necessary. Ventilation/perfusion scanning is most useful to demonstrate chronic thromboemboli (Chapter 28). **Right heart catheterization** is the definitive test for the assessment of PH, as PA pressure can be measured directly and LA pressure estimated from the pulmonary capillary wedge pressure. Patients with PH without an elevated LA pressure and no apparent pulmonary venous, lung parenchymal, chronic thromboemboli or congenital heart disease are assumed to have IPAH.

Treatment

Therapy in most patients is directed at the underlying abnormality, to relieve right ventricular strain and prevent right-sided heart failure. Hypoxaemic patients with COPD benefit from O_2 therapy to diminish hypoxic vasoconstriction. Patients with **thromboembolic disease** (Chapter 28) should receive anticoagulation and evaluation for surgical thromboembolectomy. Patients with IPAH should also receive **anticoagulation** to prevent microthrombi or the devastating effect of an acute thromboembolus (Chapter 28). There have been major advances in pharmacological therapy for PAH over the past few years. Type 5 phosphodiesterase inhibitors (e.g. sildenafil) increase cGMP and consequently augment vasorelaxation and reduce vascular remodelling. Endothelin-receptor antagonists (e.g. bosentan, dual ET_A and ET_B antagonist) block the action of endothelin-1, a potent vasoconstrictor and inducer of proliferation, the level of which correlates with PH severity. Trials have shown that both these drugs improve function, symptoms, exercise capacity and haemodynamics in PAH. Chronic infusions or nebulization of **prostacyclin** analogues improves survival, partially through vasodilatation, though effects on pulmonary vascular remodelling or endothelial function may explain its positive long-term effect. Lung transplantation is reserved for failed medical therapy.

(a) Pulmonary angiograms (A, D) and V/Q scans (B, E = ventilation scans, C, F = perfusion scans) in a healthy patient and a patient with a massive right-sided pulmonary embolism. The angiogram (D) shows complete occlusion of the right pulmonary artery. On the V/Q scan there is loss of right lung perfusion (F) but normal ventilation (E)

Normal

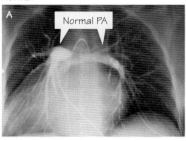

Pulmonary embolism

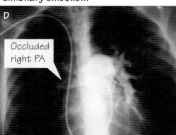

(b) Contrast CT scan showing contrast in the heart and pulmonary arteries (PA). Both the right and left PA show irregular defects, consistent with pulmonary emboli

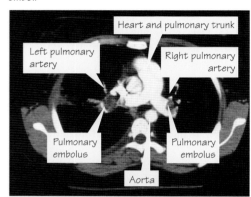

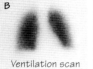

Ventilation scan

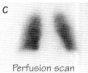

Perfusion scan

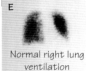

Normal right lung ventilation

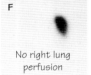

No right lung perfusion

(c) Risk factors for DVT and PE

Surgery	Hip, knee, gynaecological procedures
Trauma	Spinal trauma
General factors	Age, obesity, smoking, oral contraceptive pill (OCP)
Underlying disease	Malignancy, sepsis, stroke, autoimmune disease
Cardiovascular disease	Low flow states (e.g. cardiac failure and immobility) Vascular injury (e.g. atherosclerosis and catheters)
Inherited disorders (less common)	Deficiencies (e.g. antithrombin III, protein C and protein S) Clotting disorders (e.g. factor V leiden, antiphospholipid syndrome and dysfibrinogenaemias)

(d) DVT prophylaxis

Risk of DVT	Patient	Regime
Low (<1%)	<40 years old, minor surgery (<1 h) Minimal immobility	Early ambulation Compression stockings
Moderate (5–10%)	>40 years old, surgery (>1 h), cardiac, medical problems, CVA, hypercoagulability	Low-dose heparin (UFH or LMWH)
High (>15%)	Complicated surgery, hip or knee surgery, hip fracture, trauma	Full-dose LMWH or warfarin

LMWH = low-molecular-weight heparin
UFH = unfractionated heparin
CVA = cerebrovascular accident

Venous thromboembolism and its most significant complication, **pulmonary embolism (PE)**, are common clinical disorders that have a substantial impact on patient morbidity and mortality; Fig. 28c shows major risks. PE is most often a complication of **deep venous thrombosis (DVT)**. Both disorders are commonly underdiagnosed and require appropriate clinical suspicion and a systematic diagnostic approach. About 5 million patients develop DVT in the USA each year; approximately 500 000 subsequently develop PE and approximately 10% of these die. Prophylactic therapy in patients at risk is essential (Fig. 28d); in its absence up to 70% of patients undergoing hip or knee replacement surgery develop DVT.

Deep venous thrombosis

Nearly all clinically significant cases of PE (~90%) arise from DVT in the lower extremities, with thrombi typically originating in the calves and propagating above the knee. Approximately 15–25% will propagate into the femoral and iliac veins and have a 50% risk of embolizing to the lung. Thrombi may develop in the axillary and subclavian veins, usually due to surgery or intravenous catheters, but emboli are usually smaller, with less risk of catastrophic consequences. Soon after thrombus formation, the intrinsic fibrinolytic cascade begins to organize the thrombus. The risk of a thrombus embolizing is greatest early during ongoing proliferation and decreases once it is organized.

Pulmonary embolism

When a thrombus embolizes to the lung, respiratory or circulatory abnormalities occur due to sudden occlusion of a pulmonary artery or arteriole. Occlusion of regional perfusion causes an increase in dead space, necessitating an **increase in minute ventilation** to maintain normal $P_a CO_2$. Surfactant production distal to the embolus may be reduced after 24 hours, resulting in **atelectasis**. Hypoxaemia is common and mostly due to V_A/Q **mismatch** (Chapter 14). **Pulmonary infarction** occurs in less than 25% of cases of PE. Circulatory complications arise from obliteration of the pulmonary vascular bed and a reduction of cardiac output. Severity is related to the amount of lung embolized and the pre-existing state of the pulmonary vasculature and right ventricle (RV). A single large embolus can be catastrophic, whereas multiple small emboli can cause 'pruning' of smaller arteries. Circulatory collapse may occur with more than 50% obstruction of the pulmonary vascular bed. Less severe emboli may be fatal to patients with pre-existing lung or heart disease.

Clinical features

Clinical features of DVT are non-specific, with lower extremity pain, swelling and erythema. Homan's sign (pain in the calf on dorsiflexion of the foot) occurs in a minority of patients. Fifty per cent of DVTs are undetected.

Most patients with PE have **dyspnoea**, **pleuritic chest pain**, **haemoptysis**, **apprehension** and **tachypnoea**. With severe PE, signs related to **RV failure** (e.g. hypotension and jugular venous distension) may occur. Most patients with PE have non-specific abnormalities on chest X-ray, including atelectasis. The electrocardiogram (ECG) may show non-specific ST segment changes, and rarely, with significant RV strain, an $S_1 Q_3 T_3$ pattern (prominent S in lead I, Q and inverted T in lead III), right axis deviation (RAD) or right bundle-branch block (RBBB). **Arterial blood gas abnormalities** are common, including **widened A–a gradient**, **hypoxaemia** and **hypocapnia** (despite increased dead space).

Diagnosis

Deep venography or **pulmonary angiography** is the diagnostic standard, although **V/Q scanning** is usually the initial investigation as it is less invasive (Fig. 28a; Chapter 21). A negative perfusion scan effectively rules out PE and a 'high probability' scan (multiple segmental perfusion defects with normal ventilation) has a more than 85% probability of PE (Fig. 28a). With a high clinical suspicion, a high-probability V/Q scan has a positive predictive value of more than 95%. Unfortunately, most V/Q scans are non-diagnostic or indeterminate, with a 15–50% likelihood of PE, necessitating further imaging. **Non-invasive imaging** of the lower extremity deep veins with Doppler imaging or impedance plethysmography is useful, because the presence of thrombosis requires treatment similar to PE. In patients with underlying cardiac or pulmonary disease, **pulmonary angiography** is indicated if the above tests are non-diagnostic. Absence of DVT and a low probability V/Q scan permit treatment to be withheld. **Spiral/helical computed tomography** (CT) has a sensitivity for PE of 70–95% (higher for more proximal emboli) and a specificity of more than 90%. It also allows visualization of parenchymal abnormalities and is used in patients with chronic obstructive pulmonary disease (COPD) or extensive chest X-ray abnormalities, where V/Q scanning is indeterminate. **Echocardiography** may reveal RV dysfunction in PE and rule out **pericardial tamponade** or severe left ventricular (LV) dysfunction. **Transoesophageal echocardiography** may visualize thromboemboli in the main pulmonary arteries, but not in lobar or segmental arteries.

Treatment

The cornerstone of therapy for DVT/PE is **anticoagulation**, which stops propagation of existing thrombus and allows organization. Immediate therapy in patients with a high suspicion of PE may prevent further life-threatening embolization. Standard therapy is to give **unfractionated heparin (UFH)** or **low-molecular-weight heparin (LMWH)** for 5–7 days, followed by **warfarin** for 3–6 months. UFH and warfarin must be monitored as subtherapeutic levels increase the risk of recurrent thromboembolism. LMWH is more bioavailable and does not require monitoring. Patients with inherited or acquired hypercoagulability may require lifelong therapy.

In patients with contraindications to anticoagulation (recent surgery, haemorrhagic stroke, central nervous system metastases, active bleeding) or recurrent PE while on therapeutic anticoagulation, an **inferior vena cava (IVC) filter** may prevent fatal PE.

Although activation of **fibrinolysis** with **thrombolytics** hastens resolution of perfusion defects and RV dysfunction, convincing benefit is lacking. As thrombolytics cause increased bleeding complications, including a 0.3–1.5% risk of intracerebral haemorrhage, they are only recommended for life-threatening PE with compromised haemodynamics.

(a) CT scan of patient with Wegener's granulomatosis, showing large cavitating masses

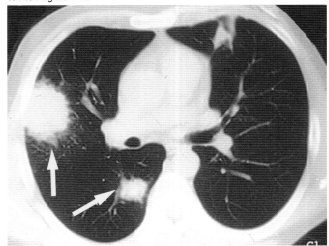

(b) Histological section showing necrobiotic regions with multinucleate giant cells (arrows)

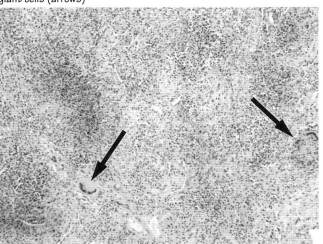

Table 1

Disease	Feature	Diagnostic antibodies	Comment
Collagen vascular disease			
Rheumatoid arthritis	Arteries		Uncommon
Scleroderma	Fibrosis in arterioles		CREST syndrome
SLE	Capillaritis		Alveolar haemorrhage
Vasculitides			
Wegener's granulomatosis	Granulomatous inflammation Arteriolar/venular vasculitis Capillaritis, fibrinoid necrosis	PR3-ANCA >> MPO-ANCA	Alveolar haemorrhage
Churg–Strauss syndrome	Necrotizing vasculitis in small arteries, arterioles and venules Granulomas, eosinophils Fibrinoid necrosis	MPO-ANCA >> PR3-ANCA	Asthma, eosinophilia
Microscopic polyangiitis	Arteriole/venule vasculitis Capillaritis, fibrinoid necrosis	MPO-ANCA > PRS-ANCA	Related to Wegener's Hepatitis B, C
Goodpasture's syndrome	Intra-alveolar haemorrhage Linear IgG in basement membrane Minimal inflammation	Anti-GBM antibodies Occassionally PR3-ANCA	Alveolar haemorrhage Smoking, recent infection
Lymphomatoid granulomatosis	Angiodestructive lymphocytes Plasma cells, atypical lymphocytes		Epstein–Barr virus Lymphoproliferative

Vasculitis is primarily associated with inflammation and necrosis of blood vessels, and includes a number of rare conditions (**vasculitides**) with high untreated mortality. Pulmonary vasculitis commonly occurs with systemic vasculitis, and may cause wheeze, hypoxaemia, pulmonary infiltrates, masses, necrotizing lesions and/or alveolar haemorrhage. Vasculitis may be secondary to systemic **collagen vascular disease** — such as **rheumatoid arthritis**, **scleroderma** or **systemic lupus erythematosus (SLE)** — or may be **primary vasculitides** that involve pulmonary blood vessels (**Wegener's granulomatosis, Churg–Strauss syndrome, microscopic polyangiitis, lymphomatoid granulomatosis** and **angiitis**). Anti-glomerular basement membrane disease (**Goodpasture's syndrome**) has a similar clinical presentation to pulmonary vasculitis.

Most primary vasculitides involve neutrophil infiltration into the lung interstitium, with consequent vascular damage by fibrinoid necrosis; capillary rupture can lead to alveolar haemorrhage. Autoantibodies against components of the cytoplasm of granulocytes and neutrophils, **anti-neutrophil cytoplasmic antibodies (ANCA)**, are diagnostic markers for vasculitis and may be part of the pathology. These are differentially characterized by neutrophil staining: cytoplasmic (c-ANCA) and peri-nuclear (p-ANCA), which are largely synonymous with PR3-ANCA (targeting peroxidase-3), and MPO-ANCA (targeting myeloperoxidase), respectively (Table 1).

Collagen vascular diseases

Rheumatoid arthritis may cause vasculitis and **pulmonary hypertension** (Chapter 27); however, this is far less frequent than pleural disease (Chapter 32) or diffuse parenchymal disease (Chapter 30). Patients may develop **Caplan's syndrome** as a result of dust inhalation (e.g. coal dust) (Chapter 33). **Limited cutaneous scleroderma** often spares lung parenchyma and causes pulmonary hypertension by direct involvement of pulmonary arterioles. While not common, **pulmonary capillaritis** causing alveolar haemorrhage secondary to **SLE** is a devastating complication with a high mortality rate. Patients generally have a pre-existing diagnosis of SLE, usually with renal involvement. Rarely, SLE may cause pulmonary hypertension by direct involvement of the pulmonary vasculature. Clinically, this is indistinguishable from **pulmonary arterial hypertension** (Chapter 27).

Vasculitides

Wegener's granulomatosis (WG) is a systemic vasculitis that predominantly involves the upper and lower respiratory systems and the renal glomeruli. Vascular inflammation may involve arterioles, capillaries and venules. Patients are generally aged 40–60 years and present with upper respiratory symptoms, usually involving the sinuses (sinusitis) or nasopharynx (ulcers, septal perforation, saddle nose deformity). Radiographic abnormalities in the chest are common, mostly as nodules or masses, often with cavitation (Fig. 29a), but they may appear as parenchymal infiltrates. Renal disease is usual and consists of glomerulonephritis with haematuria, proteinuria and red blood cell casts. Necrotizing **granulomas** (chronically inflamed tissue masses characterized by multinucleate giant cells) are seen in the lungs (Fig. 29b), nasopharynx and kidneys. WG may also involve the ears (otitis media), eyes (conjunctivitis, uveitis), heart (coronary arteries), peripheral nervous system, skin or joints. PR3-ANCA has a 60–90% sensitivity and more than 90% specificity for WG.

Churg–Strauss syndrome (*allergic granulomatosis* and *angiitis*) is a medium/small vessel granulomatous vasculitis of the lung, skin, heart,

nervous system and kidney. It is probably the second most common pulmonary vasculitis after WG. Most patients have a history of allergic rhinitis and/or asthma and peripheral eosinophilia that may predate the vasculitis by up to a decade. Patients will present with worsening asthma, fever, malaise, subcutaneous tender nodules, mononeuritis multiplex and radiographic infiltrates. There may also be pericarditis, abdominal pain and glomerulonephritis. Radiographic abnormalities are most often patchy, fleeting infiltrates, but may include cavitating nodules or masses, interstitial infiltrates or pleural effusions. CT scans may show ground glass opacities or peribronchial thickening. Lung biopsy shows perivascular granulomatous inflammation, small artery and vein vasculitis, prominent eosinophils and necrosis. The diagnosis may be made without biopsy in the presence of asthma, eosinophilia, migratory pulmonary infiltrates and neuropathy. Both PR3-ANCA and MPO-ANCA may be positive. **Treatment:** most patients respond to corticosteroids. Cyclophosphamide or azathioprine may be added in resistant cases (suppress immune system). Patients who respond to therapy seldom relapse. Patients with an onset of asthma immediately before or concurrent with vasculitis have a poorer prognosis. Overall, survival is more than 70%, with increased mortality due to cardiac, central nervous system (CNS), renal or gastrointestinal involvement.

Microscopic polyangiitis has microscopic similarities to WG and polyarteritis nodosa. In contrast to WG, MPA does not involve the nasopharynx and sinuses and is usually associated with MPO-ANCA rather than PR3-ANCA. It is often seen in patients with hepatitis B or C infection. **Treatment** with corticosteroids and cyclophosphamide substantially reduces mortality.

Goodpasture's syndrome is a facet of **anti-glomerular basement membrane** (GBM) disease, when antibodies (linear IgG) are deposited on the basement membranes of the alveoli and glomerulus, causing damage to collagen and consequent alveolar haemorrhage and glomerulonephritis, respectively. Alveolar haemorrhage occurs predominantly in smokers, or after recent respiratory infections that alter alveolar permeability. Patients present with rapidly progressive glomerulonephritis, haemoptysis, anaemia and diffuse alveolar infiltrates on radiographs. In contrast to the primary vasculitides, prolonged systemic symptoms are uncommon. Pulmonary function testing demonstrates elevated D_LCO from extravasated haemoglobin in the lung. Diagnosis requires demonstration of anti-GBM antibodies in serum or linear IgG in glomerular or alveolar basement membranes. Both PR3-ANCA and MPO-ANCA may be positive. **Treatment:** patients with Goodpasture's syndrome should be treated with high-dose corticosteroids, cyclophosphamide and sometimes plasmapheresis. Therapy may control alveolar haemorrhage, but pulmonary and renal function may not recover.

Lymphomatoid granulomatosis is a systemic vasculitis of lungs, kidneys, CNS and skin. It is strongly associated with, and may be a late complication of, **Epstein–Barr virus** infection. It behaves like an indolent lymphoproliferative disease and may transform into a B-cell lymphoma. Patients typically have fever, malaise, cough, dyspnoea and a papular rash. Radiographic abnormalities usually consist of multiple lower lobe nodular densities. Lung biopsy shows angiocentric/angiodestructive mixed cell infiltration with lymphocytes, plasma cells and atypical lymphocytes. Vascular occlusion and necrosis are common. **Treatment:** Lymphomatoid granulomatosis is considered to be a lymphoproliferative disorder and is treated with chemotherapy and corticosteroids. Without treatment, the disease progresses and is usually fatal.

30 Diffuse parenchymal (interstitial) lung diseases

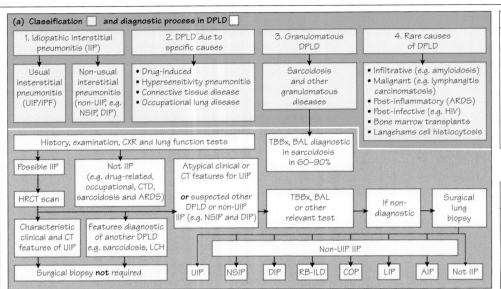

(a) Classification ▢ and diagnostic process in DPLD ▢

1. Idiopathic interstitial pneumonitis (IIP)
- Usual interstitial pneumonitis (UIP/IPF)
- Non-usual interstitial pneumonitis (non-UIP, e.g. NSIP, DIP)

2. DPLD due to specific causes
- Drug-induced
- Hypersensitivity pneumonitis
- Connective tissue disease
- Occupational lung disease

3. Granulomatous DPLD
- Sarcoidosis and other granulomatous diseases

4. Rare causes of DPLD
- Infiltrative (e.g. amyloidosis)
- Malignant (e.g. lymphangitis carcinomatosis)
- Post-inflammatory (ARDS)
- Post-infective (e.g. HIV)
- Bone marrow transplants
- Langehams cell histiocytosis

History, examination, CXR and lung function tests

Possible IIP → HRCT scan → Characteristic clinical and CT features of UIP → Surgical biopsy **not** required

Not IIP (e.g. drug-related, occupational, CTD, sarcoidosis and ARDS) → Features diagnostic of another DPLD e.g. sarcoidosis, LCH

Atypical clinical or CT features for UIP **or** suspected other DPLD or non-UIP IIP (e.g. NSIP and DIP)

TBBx, BAL diagnostic in sarcoidosis in 60–90%

TBBx, BAL or other relevant test → If non-diagnostic → Surgical lung biopsy

Non-UIP IIP: UIP | NSIP | DIP | RB-ILD | COP | LIP | AIP | Not IIP

IPF = idiopathic pulmonary fibrosis; TBBx = transbronchial biopsy; BAL = bronchoalveolar lavage; UIP = usual interstitial pneumonia; NSIP = non-specific interstitial pneumonia; DIP = desquamative interstitial pneumonia; RB = respiratory bronchiolitis; AIP = acute interstitial pneumonia; COP = organising pneumonia; LIP = lymphoctic interstitial pneumonia; DPLD = diffuse parenchymal lung disease; CTD = connective tissue disease

(b) Drug induced DPLD

Antibiotics (e.g. nitrofurantoin)
Antiarrythmias (e.g. Amiodarone and tocainide)
Anti-inflammatory (e.g. gold and penacillamine)
Anticonvulsants (e.g. dilantin)
Antihypertensives (e.g. hydralazine)
Chemotherapeutic agents (e.g. bleomycin, mitomycin C, methotrexate and busulphan)
Oxygen toxicity
Paraquat
Narcotics (inhaled or intravenous)
Therapeutic radiation

(c) Collagen vascular disease involvement in DPLD

Rheumatoid arthritis (5% but commonest cause in view of disease frequency)
Scleroderma (>70%)
Polymyositis/dermatomyostis (20–50%)
Systemic lupus erythematosus (5%)
Sjogrens syndrome (25%)
Ankylosing spondylitis (2%)

(d) HRCT scan showing subpleural honeycomb fibrosis in UIP

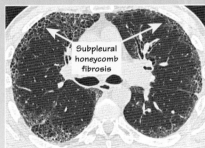

Subpleural honeycomb fibrosis

(e) HRCT scan showing subpleural sparing, coarse reticular shadowing and traction bronchiectasis in NSIP

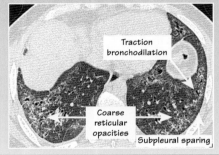

Traction bronchodilation
Coarse reticular opacities
Subpleural sparing

(f) HRCT scan showing ground glass opacification (GGO) and mosaic pattern typical of alveolitis in DIP

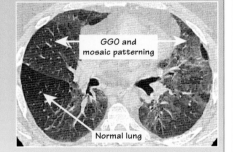

GGO and mosaic patterning
Normal lung

(g) Clinical features, age at onset, histologic pattern and radiographic features of idiopathic interstitial pneumonias

Clinical name	Age, sex	Clinical features, relation to smoking and response to treatment	Typical CT findings	CT distribution
UIP/IPF	50–80 yrs M>>F	Gradual onset. Acute exacerbations. Worse in smokers. BAL shows neutrophils (±eosinophils). Poor response to steroids and immunosuppressive agents. Median survival 2–3 years from diagnosis	Reticular abnormality + volume loss, honeycombing, traction bronchiectasis, focal GGO	Peripheral, basal + subpleural (Fig. d)
NSIP	40–50 yrs M=F	Gradual onset 6–30 months or subacute. Not related to smoking. BAL lymphocytosis. Prognosis better than UIP, especially in cellular (inflammatory) disease. Most patients improve or recover with steroid (±immunosuppressive) therapy	GGO, consolidation, reticular opacities	Peripheral, subpleural, basal (Fig. e)
COP	~55 yrs M=F	Subacute, related to CTD or lower respiratory tract infections and more common in smokers. Most patients recover with steroids but may be slow (>6 months)	Patchy consolidation and/or nodules	Subpleural, peribronchial
RB-ILD	40–50 yrs M:F 2:1	Usually occurs in heavy smokers (>30 packs a year). Characterized by pigmented intraluminal macrophages in bronchioles. Many patients improve with smoking cessation but steroid therapy may be required	Bronchial wall thickening, patchy GGO, centrilobular nodules	Diffuse
DIP	40–50 yrs M>>F	A form of severe RB-ILD. Characterized by BAL pigment-laden alveolar macrophages which fill alveolar spaces. Nearly always due to smoking. Prognosis >10 years following smoking cessation and/or steroid therapy in 70%. Progression to fibrosis in <20%.	GGO++, reticular lines	Lower zone, mainly peripheral (Fig. f)
AIP	Any age M=F	Rapidly progressive disease, indistinguishable from ARDS. Often presents after a viral URTI. No effective therapy and mortality is >50% and occurs within 4–8 weeks of onset. Recurrence or progressive fibrosis may occur in survivors.	Consolidation, GGO (lobular sparing), late traction bronchiectasis	Diffuse
LIP	Any age F>M	Often due to an underlying systemic condition (e.g. rheumatoid arthritis, systemic lupus erythematosus and myasthenia gravis). BAL lymphocytosis. Most respond to steroids but ~30% progress to diffuse fibrosis.	Centilobular nodules, GGO bronchovascular +septal thickening	Diffuse

IPF = idiopathic pulmonary fibrosis; UIP = usual interstitial pneumonia; NSIP = non-specific interstitial pneumonia; DIP = desquamative interstitial pneumonia; RB = respiratory bronchiolitis; RB-ILD = respiratory bronchiolitis-interstitial lung disease; AIP = acute interstitial pneumonia; DAD = diffuse alveolar damage; COP = cryptogenic organizing pneumonia; LIP = lymphocytic interstitial pneumonia; GGO = ground glass opacification; BAL = bronchoalveolar lavage; CTD = connective tissue disease, SLE = systemic lupus erythematosus

Diffuse parenchymal (interstitial) lung disease (DPLD/ILD) describes a group of disorders characterized by inflammation and/or fibrosis of the pulmonary interstitium (i.e. tissue between the alveolar epithelium and capillary endothelium) and the bronchovascular and septal tissues, comprising the lung's fibrous framework. Alveolar airspaces, distal airways and vasculature may also be involved.

Clinical features: Insidious onset of dyspnoea and cough, bilateral inspiratory crackles ($\pm$clubbing) and exercise-induced desaturation are common to all DPLD. Hypoxaemia and right-sided heart failure occur in advanced disease. **Pulmonary function tests** (PFT) reveal a restrictive defect with reduced total lung capacity (TLC), functional residual capacity (FRC) and residual volume (RV) due to impaired lung compliance. Gas transfer (D_LCO) is decreased due to diminished surface area for gas exchange. **Chest X-ray** (CXR) is abnormal ($>90\%$) with mainly lower lobe alveolar, interstitial or mixed infiltrates. **Bronchoalveolar lavage** (BAL) excludes other diseases (e.g. malignancy). An increase in BAL inflammatory cells indicates alveolitis and correlates with ground glass opacification (GGO) on high resolution computed tomography (HRCT) scans and may reflect rapidly progressive or potentially reversible disease. **HRCT scans** ($\pm$**histology**) are required for classification.

Classification: There are four main categories of DPLD (Fig. 30a) with considerable overlap:

1 Idiopathic interstitial pneumonitis (IIP) has two subgroups:
- *Usual interstitial pneumonia* (UIP; previously known as idiopathic pulmonary fibrosis (IPF) or cryptogenic fibrosing alveolitis), causes approximately 70% of IIP. *Pathogenesis* involves minimal inflammation with fibrosis due to fibroblast proliferation and abnormal alveolar epithelial healing. *Incidence* is approximately $5/10^5$/year. It usually occurs in older men, aged approximately 70 years. *Clinical features* include progressive dyspnoea, cough, clubbing (25–50%) and basal inspiratory crepitations interspersed with acute 'exacerbations'. *HRCT scans* show bilateral, basal and subpleural reticular changes with honeycombing and/or traction bronchiectasis (Fig. 30d). Consolidation, GGO and nodules are infrequent. *Histology* reveals peripheral, patchy damage, fibrosis and honeycombing alternating with areas of normal lung. A similar picture occurs in asbestosis, collagen vascular and drug-induced diseases. Diffuse alveolar damage (DAD) and cryptogenic organizing pneumonia (COP) occur during acute exacerbations. *Treatment:* UIP does not respond to steroids or immunosuppressants. *Median survival* from diagnosis is <3 years and worse in smokers.
- *Non-usual interstitial pneumonitis* (non-UIP) causes approximately 30% of IIP. Differences in clinical course, histology, HRCT and outcome suggest that these rare disorders are distinct clinico-pathologic entities. They include (in order of frequency) non-specific interstitial pneumonitis (NSIP), COP, previously known as bronchiolitis obliterans organising pneumonia (BOOP), acute interstitial pneumonitis (AIP; formerly known as Hamman–Rich syndrome), respiratory bronchiolitis–interstitial lung disease (RB-ILD), desquamative interstitial pneumonitis (DIP) and lymphoid interstitial pneumonitis (LIP). Clinical and radiological features, treatment response and prognosis are summarized in Fig. 30g. Presentation is earlier, mainly in men, aged 40–50 years. Pulmonary involvement is diffuse, (with subpleural sparing), less fibrotic and more cellular (Fig. 30e) than UIP. HRCT scans may show bilateral GGO, which may

be widespread, subpleural or basal (Fig. 30f). About 50% of cases are sensitive to steroid ($\pm$immunosuppressive) therapy with a median survival of >10 years. However, prognosis may be poor in steroid-resistant disease (e.g. AIP $\leq$6 months).

2 DPLD due to specific causes includes
- *Drug-induced DPLD* (Fig. 30b). Mechanisms include oxidant-mediated injury (e.g. nitrofurantoin), direct cytotoxic effects (e.g. bleomycin), cellular phospholipid deposition (e.g. amiodarone) and immune-mediated injury (e.g. hydralazine). Treatment includes drug withdrawal and occasionally steroid therapy. Irreversible damage may cause respiratory failure (e.g. amiodarone).
- *Hypersensitivity pneumonitis* (HP; also known as extrinsic allergic alveolitis) is discussed in Chapter 33. It is an inflammatory response to inhaled, mainly organic antigens, to which the patient has become sensitized (e.g. thermophilic actinomycetes in mouldy hay).
- *Connective tissue disease (CTD) DPLD* occurs in 5% of rheumatoid arthritis (RA) patients, especially those with multisystem disease (e.g. vasculitis and nodules) but is usually asymptomatic. Symptomatic DPLD occurs in many other CTD (Fig. 30c) and after some treatments (e.g. methotrexate and gold). NSIP is the predominant histological pattern except in RA, where 50% have a UIP pattern.
- *Occupational lung disease* follows inhalation of mainly mineral (e.g. coal and asbestos) dusts (Chapter 33).

3 Granulomatous DPLD: sarcoidosis, the second most frequent DPLD, and other granulomatous DPLD are discussed in Chapter 31.

4 Rare causes of DPLD include infiltrative (e.g. amyloidosis), malignant (e.g. lymphangitis carcinomatosis), post-inflammatory (e.g. ARDS and vasculitis), post-infective (e.g. HIV), bone marrow transplantation and rare lung diseases (e.g. Langerhan's cell histiocytosis).

Diagnosis (Fig. 30a): DPLD due to occupational exposure, drugs, CTD, HP or sarcoidosis is often diagnosed after a comprehensive history (i.e. occupational exposure), careful examination (e.g. for CTD), blood tests (e.g. rheumatoid factor), serology (e.g. avian precipitans), PFT and radiological imaging. In contrast, initial diagnosis of IIP is one of exclusion. Subsequent classification, to distinguish UIP from other IIP (e.g. NSIP), has important therapeutic and prognostic implications and requires an integrated clinical, radiological and pathological approach. **HRCT scans** aid differentiation. Typical clinical and HRCT features allow confident diagnosis of UIP (sensitivity 43–78%, specificity 90–97%) and avoid the need for biopsy in 50% of cases. **Surgical biopsy** is considered if radiology is not diagnostic and in non-UIP cases. Transbronchial biopsies are usually inadequate for histological classification but may be diagnostic in sarcoidosis.

Management: Treatment is considered in patients with rapidly deteriorating symptoms, inflammatory changes (e.g. GGO) or if requested despite poor evidence for benefit (e.g. UIP). **Supportive therapy** requires supplemental oxygen, pulmonary rehabilitation, nutrition, smoking cessation and palliative care. **Pharmacological therapy** includes steroids and/or immunosuppressive agents (e.g. azothioprine, methotrexate and cyclophosphamide). In steroid-sensitive conditions (e.g. COP, DIP and NSIP), a short trial of high-dose steroids may be indicated. However, in patients requiring ongoing therapy or less likely to respond (e.g. UIP), combination 'triple' therapy with low-dose prednisolone, azothioprine and N-acetylcysteine (NAC) is usually recommended. In many patients, therapy is ineffective and has significant side effects. Consider early referral for lung transplantation.

31 Sarcoidosis

(a) Causes of lung granuloma

Idiopathic: Sarcoidosis
Infective: Tuberculosis, leprosy, brucellosis, fungal, schistosomiasis, cat-scratch fever, syphilis
Malignancy: Lymphoma
Gastrointestinal: Crohn's disease, primary biliary cirrhosis
Allergic: Extrinsic allergic alveolitis
Occupational: Berylliosis, silicosis
Vasculitic: Wegener's granulomatosis, giant cell arteritis, polyarteritis nodosa, Takyasu's arteritis
Others: Thyroiditis, Langerhans' cell histiocytosis, hypogammaglobulinaemia, orchitis

(b) Causes of bihilar lymphadenopathy on CXR

Sarcoidosis

Tuberculosis

Lymphoma, leukaemia

Fungal infections (e.g. histoplasmosis)

Berylliosis

Hypogammaglobulinaenia (+recurrent infection)

(c) Characteristic CXR features in pulmonary sarcoidosis

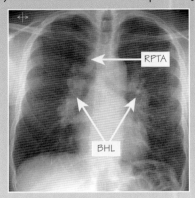

(i) Bihilar lymphadenopathy (BHL) and right paratracheal adenopathy (RPTA)

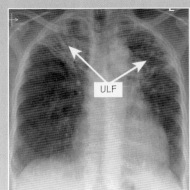

(ii) Upper lobe fibrosis (ULF)

(iii) Perihilar infiltrates

(d) Initial evaluation of sarcoidosis

History (+occupational/environmental exposure)
Examination including fundoscopy
Full blood count including lymphocyte count
Biochemistry, calcium, liver function, LDH, SACE,
  ECG, CXR, urine analysis (±calcium excretion)
Spirometry and gas transfer (DLCO)
Mantoux test (to exclude tuberculosis)

LDH = lacate dehydrogenase; SACE = serum angiotensin-converting enzyme;
ECG = electrocardiogram; CXR = chest X-ray

(e) Radiographic staging in sarcoidosis and likelihood of spontaneous resolution

Stage	Finding	Likelihood of spontaneous resolution
0	Normal chest radiograph	>90%
I	Bilateral hilar lymphadenopathy (BHL)	60–90%
II	BHL plus pulmonary infiltrates	40–60%
III	Pulmonary infiltrates (without BHL)	10–20%
IV	Pulmonary fibrosis (± bullae)	<20%

(f) CT scan of pulmonary sarcoidosis showing hilar adenopathy and peri-bronchovascular nodules. Inset shows fissural nodules/'beading' on HRCT

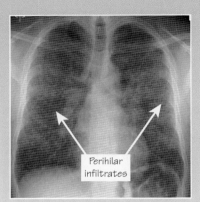

(g) Criteria for steroid therapy in sarcoidosis

Progressive symptomatic pulmonary disease
Asymptomatic pulmonary disease with ongoing loss of lung function
Cardiac disease
Neurological disease
Eye disease not responding to topical therapy
Symptomatic hypercalcaemia
Other symptomatic/progressive extrapulmonary disease

Sarcoidosis is a multisystem disorder and, although predominantly respiratory (>90%), many tissues can be affected (see below). It usually presents in young adults, 20–40 years old, and is most frequent in Afro-Caribbeans, Scandinavians, the Irish and relatives of patients with sarcoidosis. Black people are more susceptible to aggressive, systemic disease. **Incidence** varies geographically from 5 to $100/10^5$ population.

Aetiology: unknown, but it often follows exposure of a genetically susceptible person (e.g. HLA-DR) to an antigenic trigger which may be infective (e.g. mycobacteria and propionibacteria), geographical (e.g. pine pollen) or occupational (e.g. beryllium and talc). Autoimmune causes are less likely. **Histopathology** is characterized by non-caseating granulomata (NCG) and an abnormal, antigen-triggered CD4 (helper) T-cell response. Interferon-γ release stimulates granuloma formation, fibroblasts and fibrosis. Activated macrophages release serum angiotensin-converting enzyme (SACE), and B-cell stimulation produces immunoglobulin and immune complex formation. Delayed hypersensitivity (e.g. to tuberculin) is reduced due to T-cell migration. Figure 31a illustrates other causes of lung granuloma.

Clinical features: pulmonary (>90%), systemic or both:
1 Pulmonary sarcoidosis may be asymptomatic (~30%) or associated with constitutional (e.g. fever, malaise, weight loss ~30% and fatigue ~70%) and/or respiratory (e.g. non-productive cough, dyspnoea and chest discomfort ~30–50%) symptoms. Physical findings (e.g. clubbing) are rare and despite CXR infiltrates crepitations occur in less than 20% of cases. There are two distinct pulmonary presentations:

(a) *Acute sarcoidosis* (Löfgren's syndrome) occurs mainly in Caucasians with fever, erythema nodosum (EN), arthralgia, pulmonary infiltrates and bihilar lymphadenopathy (BHL; Fig. 31c(i)). The CXR findings may be asymptomatic. Exclude other causes of BHL (Fig. 31b). About 10% develop progressive lung fibrosis (Fig. 31c).

(b) *Progressive, interstitial lung disease* causes increasing dyspnoea and cough. Infiltrates ($\pm$BHL) are seen on CXR (Fig. 31c(iii)) and may progress to lung fibrosis and respiratory failure.

Diagnosis: requires a compatible clinical ($\pm$CXR) picture – histological confirmation of NCG and exclusion of other causes (e.g. TB). Figure 31d summarizes evaluation. **Disease progression** is monitored by serial clinical assessment, CXR, spirometry ($\pm D_L$CO) and SACE.

• *SACE* is raised in 80% of acute sarcoidosis and is suppressed by steroids. It aids monitoring but is not specific (i.e. raised in TB).

• *CXR* is abnormal in more than 85% of lung sarcoid, but 30–60% are asymptomatic (i.e. incidental CXR finding). BHL occurs in 50–85%, unilateral hilar lymphadenopathy in <10% and pulmonary infiltrates, usually central or in the upper lobes, in 25–50% of cases (Fig. 31c). Figure 31e shows the CXR staging system.

• *High-resolution CT scans* are not required for routine evaluation. They are useful if the CXR is normal, to discriminate between inflammation and fibrosis and to detect complications. Characteristic early features include bronchovascular micronodules (Fig. 31f), inflammation with ground glass opacification and septal thickening. Later disease causes traction bronchiectasis and fibrosis.

• *Histological confirmation* is not always needed in asymptomatic or acute disease but is recommended in symptomatic cases or if BHL is asymmetrical or massive to exclude malignancy (~10%). Transbronchial lung biopsies histologically confirm approximately 70% of cases. Bronchoalveolar lavage CD4:CD8 ratio of more than

3.5 is also specific for sarcoidosis. Tissue biopsies (e.g. skin and salivary/parotid gland) also confirm the diagnosis, but liver biopsies are not specific. A positive Mantoux test makes sarcoidosis unlikely.

• *Pulmonary function tests* (PFTs) are abnormal in 20% of stage I and 40–70% of stage II–IV radiographic disease (Fig. 31e). Typically, the defect is restrictive, but obstructive lesions occur in approximately 40% of cases. Gas transfer (D_LCO) and FVC are reduced despite a normal CXR in 15–50% of cases.

Management: Most pulmonary sarcoidosis resolves spontaneously and treatment is not required (Fig. 31e). Asymptomatic BHL and CXR infiltrates (stage II and III) should be monitored.

• *Steroid therapy* alleviates acute symptoms but does not prevent progressive pulmonary fibrosis. Figure 31g summarizes indications for treatment. The initial response to high-dose steroids (e.g. prednisolone 30–60 mg daily) is evaluated after 1–2 months and gradually tapered over 6–24 months. Relapse is common (>33% within 2 years) and is managed with prolonged low-dose steroid therapy. Prophylaxis against osteoporosis and peptic ulcers is required. Inhaled steroids have a limited role.

• *Immunosuppressive therapy* is indicated for steroid-insensitive disease and as steroid sparing agents. Methotrexate and azothioprine are beneficial in approximately 50% of steroid-resistant cases. Other cytotoxic agents include cyclophosphamide and cyclosporine. All cause toxicity and must be monitored. Hydroxychloroquine inhibits macrophage TNF-α production and granuloma formation. It is effective for hypercalcaemia, skin, lung and neurosarcoid.

• *Lung transplant* is considered in end-stage lung disease. NCG may recur in transplanted lung.

2 Extrathoracic disease is associated with fever, weight loss, malaise and arthralgia. Other features include hepatic NCG (60%), renal impairment (35%), splenomegaly, bone cysts and parotid, lacrimal or salivary gland swelling. Hypercalcaemia is common in men and Caucasians.

• *Skin* is often affected in women (~25%). EN describes painful, inflamed plaques usually on the shins. Lupus pernio (LP) produces indurated 'bluish', nose, ear or cheek lesions in chronic sarcoidosis. Topical steroids may be effective in EN, but LP requires oral steroids, hydroxychloroquine or methotrexate therapy.

• *Eye* (e.g. uveitis and scleritis) involvement is more common in women and Afro-Caribbeans (>25%). Ophthalmology assessment is essential. Treatment is with oral steroids ($\pm$ steroid eye drops).

• *Cardiac disease* (e.g. arrhythmias and heart failure) is uncommon (~5%) in the USA and Europe but causes more than 70% of sarcoid-related deaths in Japan. Treatment is with high-dose steroids, antiarrhythmics and pacemakers.

• *Neurosarcoid* (5–15% cases) causes nerve (e.g. mononeuritis multiplex) and focal cerebral (e.g. diabetes insipidus) lesions. Steroid and immunosuppressive therapy is often required.

Prognosis: factors associated with a relapsing course and poor outcome include age more than 40 years at onset, ethnic origin (e.g. Afro-Caribbean), extrathoracic disease and CXR stage (Fig. 31e). Spontaneous remission usually occurs within 3 years and failure to remit within this time predicts a chronic course (10–30%) with death in 2–5% of cases. PFT have little prognostic value, but serial FVC and D_LCO detect progressive fibrosis which accounts for 87% of sarcoid-related deaths in the USA.

32 Pleural diseases

(a) Causes of pleural effusions

Exudative (protein ratio pleural/serum >0.5 or LDH ratio pleural/serum >0.6 or pleural LDH >0.66 of top normal serum value)		Transudative (meets none of the criteria for exudative)
Infectious	**Abdominal**	Congestive heart failure
Para-pneumonic	Pancreatitis/pseudocyst	
• aerobic bacterial pneumonia	Oesophageal rupture	Cirrhosis
• anaerobic bacterial pneumonia	Liver abscess	Hepatic hydrothorax
Empyema	Splenic abscess	
Tuberculosis		Myxoedema
Parasitic	**Miscellaneous**	
• amoeba	Pulmonary embolism	Nephrotic disease
• echinococcus	Drug reactions	
• paragonimus	Asbestos exposure	Peritoneal dialysis
Viral	Haemothorax	
	Chylothorax	
Autoimmune/collagen vascular	Post-cardiac surgery	
Systemic lupus erythematosus	Post-myocardial infarction	
Rheumatoid arthritis	Meig's syndrome	
Neoplastic		
Lung cancer		
Metastatic disease		
Mesothelioma		

(b) CXR showing large pleural effusion in left lung (contrast with pneumothorax CXR in Chapter 35)

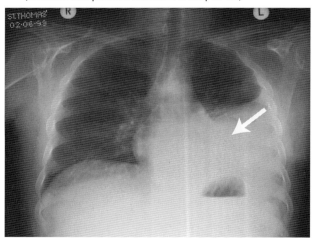

(c) CT scan demonstrating irregular (lumpy) pleural thickening of mesothelioma over lateral right chest wall (see arrows)

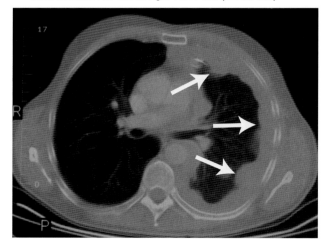

The pleurae

The potential space between the **parietal** and **visceral pleurae** serves as a coupling system between the lung and the chest wall, and normally contains a small amount of fluid. A negative pleural pressure is maintained by the dynamic tension between the chest wall and the lung (Chapter 3). Both pleurae have a systemic blood supply and lymphatics, although lymphatic drainage of the pleural space is predominantly via the parietal pleura. Fluid flux through the pleural space is determined by Starling's relationship between microvascular pressures, oncotic pressures, permeability and surface area. Normally, there is net filtration of **transudative** (protein-poor) fluid into the pleural space that is balanced by resorption via the parietal lymphatics.

Pneumothorax is an important condition that occurs when air enters the pleural space and pleural pressure rises to atmospheric pressure; pneumothorax is discussed in detail in Chapter 35.

Chylothorax is due to accumulation of triglyceride-rich lymph in the pleural space, generally as the result of damage to the thoracic duct causing leakage into the pleural space, for example due to trauma or carcinoma.

Empyema is accumulation of pus.

Pleurisy is a term commonly used to describe the sharp localized pain arising from any disease of the pleura. It is made worse by deep inspiration and coughing.

Pathophysiology

Most diseases of the pleura present with **pleural effusion**, which can be detected on chest X-ray (CXR) when more than 300 mL of fluid is present (Fig. 32b). Effusions are due to excessive fluid formation or inadequate fluid clearance. Symptoms develop if the fluid is **inflammatory** or if **pulmonary mechanics** are compromised. Thus, the most common symptoms of a pleural effusion are **pleuritic chest pain**, **dull aching pain**, **fullness of the chest** or **dyspnoea**. Physical examination reveals decreased breath sounds, dullness to percussion, decreased tactile or vocal fremitus. If there is inflammation, there may be a friction rub. **Compressive atelectasis** (partial lung collapse) may cause bronchial breath sounds.

It is useful to categorize pleural effusions as **transudative** or **exudative** (Fig. 32a).

Transudative effusions are usually due to an imbalance in Starling's forces across normal pleural membranes, have protein-poor fluid, are often bilateral and are not associated with fever, pleuritic pain or tenderness to palpation. The most common cause of a transudative effusion is **congestive heart failure**. Other causes include cirrhosis with ascites, nephrotic syndrome, pericardial disease or peritoneal dialysis.

Exudative effusions imply disease of the pleura or the adjacent lung and are characterized by an increased protein, lactate dehydrogenase (LDH), cholesterol or white blood cell count (WBC) (Fig. 32a). The differential diagnosis of exudative effusions is broad, including infection, malignancy, autoimmune disease, oesophageal perforation and pancreatitis.

Diagnostic evaluation of pleural effusion should include measurement of pleural aspirate cell count with differential, pH, protein, LDH, cholesterol and glucose. These studies usually distinguish exudates from transudates and will often suggest a specific diagnosis. For example, extremely low glucose is typical for empyema, malignancy, tuberculosis (Chapter 38), rheumatoid arthritis, systemic lupus erythematosus (SLE) or oesophageal perforation. If clinically indicated, a specific diagnosis may be obtained from microbiological stains and culture, cytopathology, amylase, triglycerides and measurement of antinuclear antibody (ANA) titre. Although all patients with SLE have a positive ANA titre in the pleural fluid, it is also present in a significant proportion (~15%) of other effusions; these may be related to malignancy.

Treatment is for the underlying condition, but persistent or reaccumulating effusions can be drained to dryness (slowly so as to avoid severe pain).

Specific conditions

Pneumonia (Chapters 36 and 37) commonly causes parapneumonic pleural effusions. These effusions are usually sterile exudates with a neutrophilic leukocytosis and require only treatment of the pneumonia to resolve. However, if bacteria invade the pleural space, a complicated parapneumonic effusion or empyema will develop. These effusions are characterized by a low pH and extensive fibrin deposition causing fluid loculation and require adequate open or closed drainage for healing. *Streptococcus pneumoniae*, *Staphylococcus aureus*, Gram-negative bacteria and anaerobes commonly cause complicated effusions.

Tuberculosis pleurisy occurs when a subpleural focus of primary infection ruptures into the pleural space, causing a delayed hypersensitivity response. Subsequently, an exudative effusion with a lymphocytic leukocytosis, a paucity of macrophages and an elevated adenosine deaminase will develop. Patients develop fever, dyspnoea, pleuritic pain and a positive tuberculin response (Chapter 38). Granulomatous inflammation is seen on pleural biopsy, and culture of pleural tissue has the highest diagnostic yield.

Primary lung malignancies or **metastases** to the lung may cause pleural effusions by direct invasion or by obstruction of parietal lymphatic drainage. Malignant effusions are mostly exudative (90%), often with a very high LDH, low pH and low glucose. Cytology of the pleural fluid has a high diagnostic yield. Symptomatic pleural effusions may respond to therapy for the underlying malignancy, although palliative obliteration of the pleural space (**pleurodesis**) is often necessary to relieve dyspnoea or chest pain.

Mesothelioma is an uncommon malignancy that originates in the pleura and/or peritoneum (Chapter 33). Over 75% of cases develop 20–30 years after occupational asbestos exposure. Asbestos may also cause benign pleural effusions or calcified plaques on the parietal pleura in the lower lungs or along the diaphragmatic surface. Mesothelioma typically develops in men aged 50–70 years, presenting with insidious dyspnoea and aching chest pain. CXRs usually show unilateral pleural effusion (Fig. 32b), and computed tomography (CT) shows lumpy fibrotic encasement of the pleural space (Fig. 32c). Pleural fluid cytology is not usually diagnostic. Thoracoscopic biopsies have the highest yield. Treatment is generally palliative, including pleurodesis. The prognosis is poor, with a median survival of approximately 1 year.

33 Occupational and environmental-related lung disease

(a) Common examples of irritant gases and other agents causing lung-specific responses

Agent	Source	Response
Ammonia	Industrial refrigeration leaks, fertilizers	**Low exposure** Exacerbations of asthma and COPD Enhanced response to allergen
Chlorine gas	Industrial leakage, water purification including swimming pools, household bleach (liquid/powder) interactions	**Moderate exposure** Mild mucosal irritation Airway inflammation and bronchiolitis
Hydrogen sulphide	Sewers and manure pits, fossil fuel extraction	**Severe exposure**
Nitrogen dioxide Nitrogen oxides	Vehicle exhausts, welding, power stations, oil refineries, gas and oil burning equipment, organic decomposition, structural or polymer fires	Epithelial damage leading to diffuse alveolar damage Pulmonary oedema and ARDS
Ozone	Vehicle exhausts, welding, copiers, ozone generators, bleaching, water treatment, plasma welding	**In some cases – late response (2–8 weeks)** Bronchiolitis obliterans after initial recovery
Sulphur dioxide	Combustion of fossil fuels, power stations, oil refineries, smelters, oil burning heaters, mining, ore refining, cement manufacturing, refrigeration plants	**Also**: direct bronchoconstriction, especially in asthmatics
Acrolein, aldehydes	Structural or wildland fires, other combustion	**Also**: strongly pro-inflammatory (esp. acrolein)
Diesel particulates (<10 μm)	Diesel engines	Airway/alveolar inflammation Increased deaths in elderly
Heavy metals (cadmium, mercury)	Welding, brazing, metal cutting, metal reclamation	Acute pneumonitis 12–24 hours after exposure
Paraquat	Ingestion of herbicides	Accelerated, chemically induced pulmonary fibrosis
Polycyclic hydrocarbons Hydrocarbons	Diesel exhaust, tobacco smoke Ingestion of hydrocarbons (children)	Cancer Aspiration hydrocarbon pneumonitis

(b) Typical causes of allergic alveolitis

Disease/occupation	Material	Causative agent
Farmer's lung	Mouldy hay or other vegetable matter	Thermophilic actinomycetes bacteria (*Saccharopolyspora rectivirgula, Thermoactinomyces* species)
Bagassosis	Sugarcane	
Mushroom workers	Compost	
Humidifier fever	Contaminated water	– Also *Klebsiella oxytoca*, amoebae
Pigeon fancier's (breeder's) lung	Feathers and excreta	Avian proteins
Farmers, sawmill, tobacco, esparto grass and brewery workers	Fungal contamination of materials	Primarily *Aspergillus* species
Cheese, laboratory, cork workers	Fungal contamination of materials	Primarily *Penicillium* species
Household	Fungal infestations of damp walls and woodwork	Multiple fungal species
– other bacterial causes	Contamination of water, wood shavings, etc.	*Bacillus subtilis, Klebsiella, Epicoccum nigrum*, non-tubercular mycobacteria

The most common form of occupational and environmental lung disease is **asthma** (Chapters 24 and 25). The UK government has reported that 750 000 people with asthma work in an environment that triggers their symptoms, and more than 3000 per year develop asthma as a result of workplace substances. While the most common cause of occupational asthma is isocyanates (e.g. paint and plastics), grain and flour dust are not far behind, and secondary smoking is most commonly reported to exacerbate symptoms. It is estimated that elimination of occupational asthma alone could have a benefit of up to £1 billion over 10 years; education and prevention are therefore key targets. Atmospheric pollution in the form of car exhausts, diesel particulates and smoke, particularly by main roads and in cities, exacerbates symptoms of respiratory disease and can lead to increased mortality in the vulnerable and elderly.

Response to acute lung irritants

Inhaled irritants (Fig. 33a) cause exacerbation of asthma and chronic obstructive pulmonary disease (COPD), coughing and dyspnoea through activation of irritant receptors (Chapter 12), and irritation of mucous membranes. Highly soluble agents (e.g. ammonia and sulphur dioxide) cause immediate irritation in the upper airways, whereas less soluble agents (e.g. chlorine and ozone) favour deeper penetration to alveolar epithelial cells, which are particularly susceptible to injury. High concentrations lead to extensive lung injury, primarily by damage to epithelium, consequent inflammation and **pulmonary oedema**. Development of **acute respiratory distress syndrome** (ARDS) is common, and treatment is similar (Chapter 41). Some patients who initially recover from moderate or severe exposure may subsequently develop **bronchiolitis obliterans** (obliteration of bronchioles by fibrous growth) after 2–8 weeks. Although steroids may slow progression, prognosis is often poor.

Inhalation of mineral dusts (pneumoconiosis)

Coal worker's pneumoconiosis (CWP) is caused by inhalation of coal or carbon dust. In **simple CWP**, the upper lobes of the lung contain small (<4 mm), round opacities (coal macules) consisting of dust, dust-laden macrophages and fibroblasts. These may enlarge to fibrosed coal nodules. Weakening of bronchiolar walls leads to focal emphysema, which together with macules is characteristic of CWP. Simple CWP is often described as symptomless, with no change in lung function. It can however develop into **progressive massive fibrosis** (PMF), with black fibrotic masses from 1 cm to several centimetres in diameter, which may have necrotic cavities. Obliteration and disruption of airways result in emphysema. Patients show irreversible airflow limitation, loss of lung volume and elastic recoil, and reduced $D_{L}CO$, with breathlessness on exertion. Treatment is limited, and similar to other progressive fibrotic diseases (Chapter 25). **Caplan's syndrome** is a nodular form of CWP associated with the defective immunology of rheumatoid disease; it may also occur with asbestosis or silicosis.

Asbestos is a fibrous mixture of silicates that is highly resistant to degradation. The fibres are 1–2 μm wide, but up to 50 μm (**blue asbestos** – crocidolite) or 2 cm (**white asbestos** – chrysotile) long. They are thus easily trapped in the lung. Blue asbestos is far more dangerous. Regulations have reduced exposure since the 1980s, but the presence of asbestos in buildings and the long interval between exposure and disease development mean that asbestos-related disease will be encountered for some time. **Asbestos bodies** (protein-covered fibres) in the lungs are indicative of exposure, but not disease. The type and extent of disease largely depend on exposure. **Asbestosis** is a fibrous lung disease developing up to 10 years after heavy exposure. Patients present with progressive dyspnoea, basal crackles on inspiration and sometimes finger clubbing. There is a restrictive lung function defect and reduced $D_{L}CO$, with diffuse streaky shadows on X-ray and thickening of visceral pleura; **honeycomb lung** is often prominent in the lower lobes. Prognosis is poor. **Mesothelioma** (Chapter 32) can develop up to 40 years after light exposure, and is invariably fatal. Milder forms of asbestos-induced pleural disease produce dyspnoea and restrictive defects coupled with pleural thickening and plaques or effusions, with scattered fibrotic foci. No treatment is effective for asbestos-related disease, as the stimulus remains in the lungs. Asbestos-related lung cancer is discussed in Chapter 40.

Silicosis is a fibrotic disease caused by inhalation of silica, with a low prevalence in developed nations. Occupations at risk include mining, stone-working, manufacture of abrasives, foundry work and glass-working. Silica is very toxic to macrophages and thus highly fibrogenic. Chronic silicosis (over decades) is characterized by **silicotic nodules** of collagen around a cell-free core, first developing in hilar lymph nodes. In acute silicosis due to heavy exposure, severe dyspnoea may develop over months. The clinical features of silicosis are similar to PMF.

Inhalation of organic material

Extrinsic allergic alveolitis (or **hypersensitivity pneumonitis**) is a diffuse inflammatory disease of small airways and alveoli caused by allergens, primarily microbial spores, that are small enough to reach the alveoli (Fig. 33b). The most common example is **farmer's lung**, caused by dust from mouldy hay or plants contaminated with **thermophilic actinomycetes** bacteria, which thrive in warm moist conditions. Typically, symptoms occur several hours after exposure, and include fever, dyspnoea and cough. Although early removal of exposure results in rapid recovery, continuous exposure leads to progressive **interstitial fibrosis** (Chapter 32), with infiltration of inflammatory cells and formation of **granulomas** (chronically inflamed tissue masses characterized by multinucleate giant cells, see Fig. 29b). Patients present with dyspnoea, restrictive defects and decreased $D_{L}CO$. Fluffy nodular shadowing or ground glass opacity may be shown in CXR, with honeycomb lung (Chapter 32) in severe cases. Detailed histories are required to establish antigens, with confirmation by precipitating antibodies in serum. **Management** centres on abolishing antigen exposure. High-dose corticosteroids can regress early disease, but established disease with fibrosis is irreversible and can progress to respiratory failure. **Differential diagnosis** includes asthma (Chapters 24 and 25), sarcoidosis (Chapter 31), viral and mycoplasma pneumonias (Chapters 36 and 37) and mycobacterial infections.

Byssinosis occurs in workers handling raw cotton, flax and hemp. It is characterized by chest tightness, cough and/or shortness of breath on the first day back at work, with recovery as the week progresses. It is primarily due to acute bronchoconstriction, possibly related to contaminating bacterial endotoxins. Long-term exposure causes a disease similar to chronic bronchitis (Chapter 26), with chronic productive cough, progressive decline in lung function and disability.

(a) Mean survival of CF patients

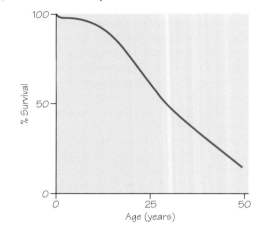

(b) Development of respiratory problems in CF

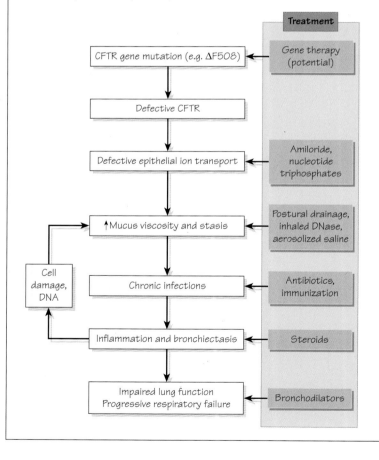

(c) Other conditions associated with CF

Condition	% of CF patents
Delayed development, puberty	100%
Male infertility (absent/obstructed vas deferens and epididymis)	98%
Female infertility	20%
Pancreatic insufficiency	85%
Nasal polyps	15–20%, most in 2nd decade
Symptomatic sinusitis	10% children 25% adults
Rectal prolapse	20% children Rare in adults
Bone demineralization (vitamin D deficiency)	Common
Hypertrophic osteoarthropathy	15% adults
Dysfunctional gallbladder or gallstones	10–30%
Biliary cirrhosis	5% adults

(d) Some conditions associated with bronchiectasis

Allergic bronchopulmonary aspergillosis (Chapter 33)
α_1-Antitrypsin deficiency (Chapters 18, 26)
Bronchial obstruction (foreign bodies, mucus, tumour)
Congenital cartilage deficiency (Williams–Campbell syndrome)
Cystic fibrosis
Fibrotic disease and alveolitis (Chapters 30 and 33)
HIV and immunodeficiency (Chapter 39)
Infection (e.g. measles and pertussis), pneumonia (Chapters 36 and 37)
Lung transplant
Primary ciliary dyskinesia (Kartagener's syndrome, Chapter 18)
Rheumatoid arthritis
Tuberculosis (Chapter 38)
Tracheobronchomegaly (Mounier–Kuhn syndrome)

Cystic fibrosis (CF) is the primary cause of severe chronic lung disease in children, although 90% of children now survive into their second decade (Fig. 34a). CF is characterized by **chronic bronchopulmonary infection** and airway obstruction (Fig. 34b) and by **exocrine pancreatic insufficiency** with consequent effects on gut function, nutrition and development. The key feature of CF is **increased viscosity** and **subsequent stasis of epithelial mucus**. There is usually an **increased salt content of sweat**. Figure 34c shows some associated disorders.

CF is an **autosomal recessive trait** that is the most common genetic cause of morbidity and mortality in the white population, with a prevalence of approximately 1 in 2000 live births; nearly 5% of white people of European descent are heterozygous carriers. Prevalence is far less in others, being approximately 1 in 17 000 for those of African descent. CF is due to mutations in a gene on chromosome 7 encoding for the **cystic fibrosis transmembrane conductance regulator** (CFTR), a cyclic adenosine monophosphate (cAMP)-regulated epithelial chloride channel that can also alter activity of other ionic transporters. Dysfunction of CFTR impairs epithelial chloride, sodium and water transfer and thus causes **reduced mucus hydration** and **increased viscosity** (Chapter 18). Over 800 mutations in the CFTR gene have been described, but the most common, found in approximately 65% of patients with CF, is deletion of the phenylalanine codon at position 508, the **ΔF508** mutation.

Clinical features

The lungs of neonates with CF are often normal, but rapid development of respiratory symptoms, including refractory cough and infections, is usual. CF patients nearly always have an increased lung volume and **finger clubbing** (increased curvature of the nail and loss of normal angle between nail and nail bed) (Chapter 19). Recurrent bronchopulmonary infections, primarily as a result of defective mucus clearance, are rarely cleared once established and eventually result in **bronchiectasis** (see below), extensive lung damage and dysfunction. Spontaneous **pneumothorax** (Chapter 35) and **haemoptysis** (spitting blood; Chapter 45) are not uncommon. About 10% of neonates present with meconium ileus (failure to pass meconium), which can cause death in the first day of life; 20% of older patients exhibit a similar ileal obstruction (**meconium ileus equivalent**, MIE). Eighty-five per cent of patients have steatorrhoea (high fat stools) as a result of pancreatic insufficiency. Some patients have only mild respiratory symptoms for many years, but this is inevitably followed by a characteristic increase in the frequency and severity of periods of exacerbation of symptoms (cough, dyspnoea, loss of appetite). Eventually, severe restrictions in activity herald the end-stage disease, followed by respiratory failure, hypoxaemia, pulmonary hypertension and death.

Diagnosis

Several factors need to be taken into account, including a **family history** of the disease and the presence of typical respiratory and gastrointestinal disorders (Fig. 34c). A **sweat chloride** or **sodium** concentration above 60 mmol/L is diagnostic when coupled with such disorders, although approximately 1% of CF patients may have normal sweat electrolytes. DNA analysis can detect known mutations (e.g. ΔF508), but is limited by the high number of unknown mutations. In later disease, chest X-rays can detect bronchiectasis (see below). Neonates can be screened for CF by blood immunoreactive trypsin, which can detect many, but not all cases.

Management

The primary objectives of treatment are to **control infection, promote mucus clearance** and **improve nutrition**. Early antibiotic therapy is crucial to inhibit progression of the disease. Choice of antibiotic is determined following identification of infecting organisms. The dosage should be higher in CF patients and the course longer. Development of resistance is a key problem and is transferable; segregation of patients is thus advisable. Adequate immunization for measles, pertussis and influenza is important, as these organisms are particularly dangerous in CF.

Clearance: Training by physiotherapists in postural drainage (tipping the body so that the infected lobe is uppermost) is vital, coupled with chest percussion to mobilize secretions to the upper airways where they can be coughed up. Such treatment is prescribed one to four times a day. Recently introduced therapies include inhalation of DNase, an enzyme that breaks down DNA from dead cells, which contributes to mucus viscosity. Inhalation of aerosolized saline may improve mucus hydration, as may blockade of sodium reabsorption with amiloride or stimulation of chloride secretion with nucleotide triphosphates. Cough should never be suppressed, as it is an important method of clearance.

Other therapies: Bronchodilators (β-agonists) may improve lung function, and corticosteroids may assist inflammation in some patients. A potential therapy under intense investigation is gene transfer of the normal CFTR gene. In end-stage respiratory disease, a lung transplant should be considered.

Nutrition: Most patients with CF require pancreatic enzymes with meals, supplemented with vitamins. High-calorific foods should be advised.

Bronchiectasis

Bronchiectasis is an abnormal and permanent dilatation of proximal (>2 mm) bronchi due to inflammation and subsequent destruction of the elastic and muscular components of their walls (Chapter 44). It is normally associated with defects in **mucociliary clearance** (Chapter 18) and **persistent respiratory infections**. Onset is often in childhood, following pulmonary infections complicating measles or pertussis. Since the introduction of antibiotics, the most common cause of bronchiectasis is now CF (Fig. 34d), except in poorly resourced countries. Symptoms depend on the severity and location of diseased bronchi, but commonly include persistent productive cough, with large quantities of foul-smelling purulent sputum as the disease worsens. Severity has been correlated with the volume of sputum produced, but not with dyspnoea. Haemoptysis and recurrent pneumonia or abscesses are common; haemoptysis is normally mild, but can become life-threatening, particularly in CF patients. Fever, anaemia and weight loss may accompany the disease. Patients often develop finger clubbing, metastatic abscesses, respiratory failure and amyloidosis. Chest X-rays and high-resolution computed tomography (HRCT) can often detect the dilated and thickened bronchi (Chapter 45). **Management** is similar to that for CF, although without the nutritional requirements.

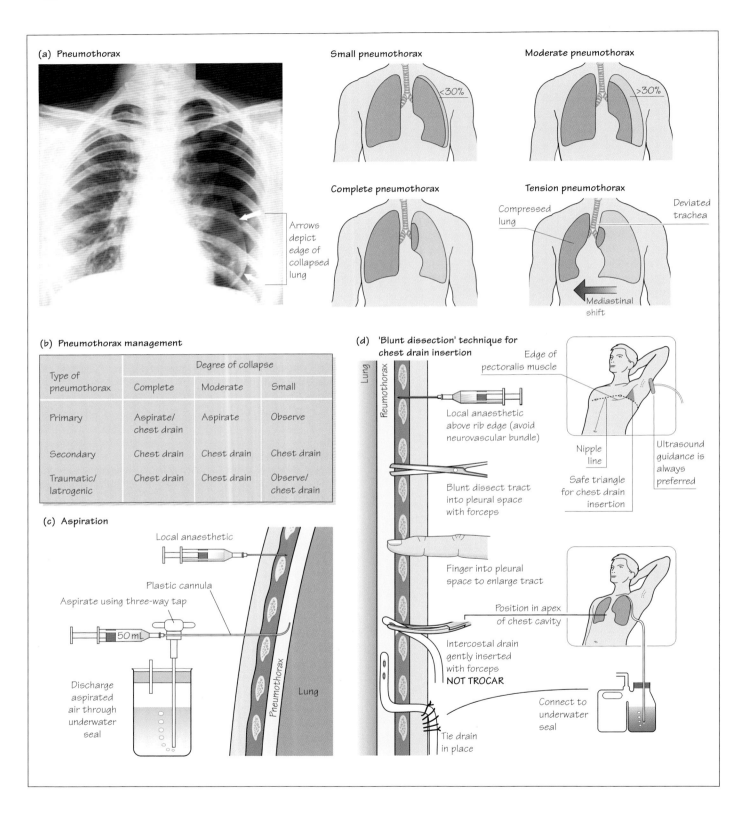

(a) Pneumothorax

Arrows depict edge of collapsed lung

Small pneumothorax
<30%

Moderate pneumothorax
>30%

Complete pneumothorax

Tension pneumothorax
Compressed lung
Deviated trachea
Mediastinal shift

(b) Pneumothorax management

Type of pneumothorax	Degree of collapse		
	Complete	Moderate	Small
Primary	Aspirate/ chest drain	Aspirate	Observe
Secondary	Chest drain	Chest drain	Chest drain
Traumatic/ Iatrogenic	Chest drain	Chest drain	Observe/ chest drain

(c) Aspiration

Local anaesthetic

Plastic cannula

Aspirate using three-way tap

50 mL

Discharge aspirated air through underwater seal

Pneumothorax

Lung

(d) 'Blunt dissection' technique for chest drain insertion

Lung
Pneumothorax

Local anaesthetic above rib edge (avoid neurovascular bundle)

Blunt dissect tract into pleural space with forceps

Finger into pleural space to enlarge tract

Intercostal drain gently inserted with forceps
NOT TROCAR

Tie drain in place

Edge of pectoralis muscle

Nipple line

Safe triangle for chest drain insertion

Ultrasound guidance is always preferred

Position in apex of chest cavity

Connect to underwater seal

A pneumothorax is a collection of air between the visceral and parietal pleura causing a real rather than potential pleural space. Recognition and early drainage can be lifesaving. Predisposing and precipitating factors include necrotizing lung pathology, chest trauma, ventilator-associated lung injury and cardiothoracic surgery.

Pneumothorax classification
Primary spontaneous pneumothorax (PSP)
This is caused by rupture of small apical subpleural air cysts ('blebs') but rarely causes significant physiological disturbance. Tall young (20–40 years old) men (male/female 5:1) with no underlying lung disease are usually affected. It is the most common type of pneumothorax (prevalence $8/10^5$ per year, rising to $200/10^5$ per year in subjects >1.9 m in height). Following a second primary spontaneous pneumothorax (PSP), recurrence is likely ($>60\%$). Pleurodesis to fuse the visceral and parietal pleura using medical (e.g. pleural insertion of bleomycin or talc) or surgical (e.g. abrasion of the pleural lining) means is recommended.

Secondary pneumothorax
This is associated with respiratory diseases that damage lung architecture, most commonly obstructive (e.g. chronic obstructive pulmonary disease (COPD) and asthma), fibrotic or infective (e.g. pneumonia), and occasionally rare or inherited disorders (e.g. Marfan's and cystic fibrosis). The incidence of secondary pneumothorax (SP) increases with age and the severity of the underlying lung disease. These patients usually require hospital admission as even a small SP in a patient with reduced respiratory reserve may have more serious implications than a large PSP. ICU patients with lung disease are at particular risk of SP due to the high pressures ('barotrauma') and alveolar overdistention ('volutrauma') associated with mechanical ventilation. 'Protective' ventilation strategies using low-pressure, limited volume ventilation reduce this risk.

Traumatic (iatrogenic) pneumothorax
This follows blunt (e.g. road traffic accidents) or penetrating (e.g. fractured ribs and stab wounds) chest trauma. Therapeutic procedures (e.g. line insertion and thoracic surgery) are common causes of iatrogenic pneumothorax.

Tension pneumothorax
A **tension pneumothorax** may complicate PSP or SP but is most common during mechanical ventilation and following traumatic pneumothorax. It occurs when air accumulates in the pleural cavity faster than it can be removed. Increased intrathoracic pressure causes mediastinal shift, compression of functioning lung, inhibition of venous return and shock due to reduced cardiac output. It is a medical emergency and fatal if not rapidly relieved by drainage. Detection is a clinical diagnosis; awaiting chest X-ray (CXR) confirmation may be life-threatening. Immediate drainage with a 14G needle in the second intercostal space in the midclavicular line is essential. A characteristic 'hiss' of escaping gas confirms the diagnosis. A chest drain is then inserted.

Clinical assessment
Pneumothorax is graded and treated according to Fig. 35a and Table b. Sudden breathlessness and/or sharp pleuritic pain suggests a pneumothorax. Most PSPs are small ($<30\%$) and cause few symptoms other than pain. Clinical signs can be surprisingly difficult to detect, but in larger pneumothoraxes reduced air entry and hyperresonant percussion over one hemithorax are characteristic and may be associated with tachypnoea and cyanosis. Cardiorespiratory compromise may develop remarkably quickly in a tension pneumothorax and requires immediate drainage. Occasionally, other pulmonary air leaks may occur (see below). **Monitoring** reveals tachycardia, hypotension and desaturation. **Blood gases** may demonstrate respiratory failure. **CXR** confirms the diagnosis (Fig. 35a). **Computed tomography (CT) scan** may detect localized pneumothoraxes.

Management
Immediate supportive therapy includes supplemental oxygen and analgesia. Treatment is dependent on the cause, size and symptoms.

A tension pneumothorax must be drained immediately. A small PSP ($<30\%$) is simply observed and spontaneous reabsorption is confirmed on serial outpatient CXR. A PSP $>30\%$ may be aspirated through a 16G needle in the second intercostal space in the midclavicular line, using a 50 mL syringe connected to a three-way tap and underwater seal (Fig. 35c). Following overnight observation, successful aspiration is confirmed by lung re-expansion on repeat CXR. Occasionally, intercostal tube drainage is required for a large PSP with respiratory failure or if aspiration is unsuccessful.

In general, SP and traumatic pneumothoraxes *always* require hospital admission and intercostal chest drain insertion (Fig. 35d). Multiple intercostal drains may be needed to ensure adequate lung re-expansion in some patients with multiple loculated pneumothoraxes. In mechanically ventilated patients, high airway pressures or large tidal volumes encourage persistent leaks and must be avoided.

Small chest drains (16 G) are nearly always adequate. Large chest drains are painful and have no significant benefits.

A persistent drain leak suggests development of a **bronchopleural fistula** (BPF). High flow, wall suction with pressures of 5–50 cmH$_2$O, may oppose visceral and parietal pleura, allowing spontaneous pleurodesis. Physiotherapy and bronchial toilette are required to maintain airway patency. Early advice on surgical BPF management is essential. Video-assisted thoracoscopy is as effective as thoracotomy at correcting BPF but causes less respiratory dysfunction.

Chest drains are removed when CXR confirms lung expansion and there has been no air leakage through the drain for more than 24 hours. Drains should not be clamped before removal. Following adequate analgesia, the drain is pulled out when the patient is in inspiration. Purse string sutures around the drainage site are then tightly secured.

Air leaks
Pneumomediastinum describes air in the mediastinal–pleural reflection, outlining the heart and great vessels on CXR. Air may also dissect along perivascular sheaths into the neck, causing **subcutaneous emphysema (SE)** or around the heart with **pneumopericardium**, which may cause tamponade. Air leaks follow traumatic damage to the trachea, bronchus and oesophagus or ventilator-induced barotrauma. SE may cause localized cervical or grotesque facial and body swelling. It has a characteristic crackling sensation on palpation. The voice may have a nasal quality, and auscultation over the precordium may reveal a 'crunch' with each heart beat (Homan's sign). Management includes good drainage of pneumothorax and 'protective' ventilation strategies (Chapter 42). Failure of spontaneous resolution should prompt investigation, including bronchoscopy, for problems that decrease chest drain efficiency or undetected air leaks.

(a) Pneumonia affecting the right lower lobe

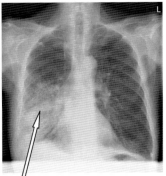

Consolidation right lower lobe

(b) Pneumonia affecting lingula lobe

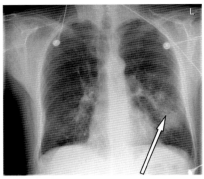

Consolidation lingula lobe

Table 2. Risk factors for pneumonia

Age: >65, <5 years old
Chronic disease (e.g. renal and lung)
Diabetes mellitus
Immunosuppression (e.g. drugs and HIV)
Alcohol dependency
Aspiration (e.g. epilepsy)
Recent viral illness (e.g. influenza)
Malnutrition
Mechanical ventilation
Postoperative (e.g. obesity and smoking)
Environmental (e.g. psittacosis)
Occupational (e.g. Q fever)
Travel abroad (e.g. paragonimiasis)
Air conditioning (e.g. Legionella)

Table 1. Microorganisms and pathological insults that cause pneumonia

Bacterial infections	Atypical infections	Fungal infection
Streptococcus pneumoniae	Mycoplasma pneumoniae	Aspergillus
Haemophilus influenzae	Legionella pneumophila	Histoplasmosis
Klebsiella pneumoniae	Coxiella burnetii	Candida
Pseudomonas aeruginosa	Chlamydia psittaci	Nocardia
Gram-negative (E. coli)		
Viral infections	**Protozoal infections**	**Other causes**
Influenza	Pneumocystis carinii	Aspiration
Coxsackie	Toxoplasmosis	Lipoid pneumonia
Adenovirus	Amoebiasis	Bronchiectasis
Respiratory syncytial	Paragonimiasis	Cystic fibrosis
Cytomegalovirus		Radiation

(c) Non-hospital (i.e. community) management of CAP using the recently validated CRB-65 score

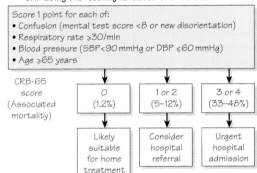

Score 1 point for each of:
- Confusion (mental test score <8 or new disorientation)
- Respiratory rate >30/min
- Blood pressure (SBP<90 mmHg or DBP ≤60 mmHg)
- Age ≥65 years

CRB-65 score (Associated mortality)	0 (1.2%)	1 or 2 (5–12%)	3 or 4 (33–48%)
	Likely suitable for home treatment	Consider hospital referral	Urgent hospital admission

(e) Complications and infection specific features of pneumonia

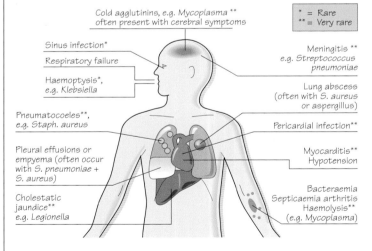

Cold agglutinins, e.g. Mycoplasma **
often present with cerebral symptoms

* = Rare
** = Very rare

Sinus infection*

Respiratory failure

Haemoptysis*, e.g. Klebsiella

Pneumatocoeles**, e.g. Staph. aureus

Pleural effusions or empyema (often occur with S. pneumoniae + S. aureus)

Cholestatic jaundice** e.g. Legionella

Meningitis ** e.g. Streptococcus pneumoniae

Lung abscess (often with S. aureus or aspergillus)

Pericardial infection**

Myocarditis** Hypotension

Bacteraemia Septicaemia arthritis Haemolysis** (e.g. Mycoplasma)

(d) Management of CAP in patients admitted to hospital using the recently validated CURB-65 score

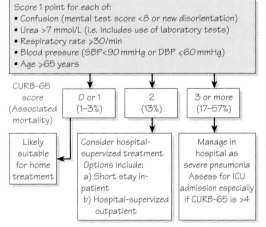

Score 1 point for each of:
- Confusion (mental test score <8 or new disorientation)
- Urea >7 mmol/L (i.e. includes use of laboratory tests)
- Respiratory rate >30/min
- Blood pressure (SBP<90 mmHg or DBP ≤60 mmHg)
- Age ≥65 years

CURB-65 score (Associated mortality)	0 or 1 (1–3%)	2 (13%)	3 or more (17–57%)
	Likely suitable for home treatment	Consider hospital-supervized treatment Options include: a) Short stay in-patient b) Hospital-supervised outpatient	Manage in hospital as severe pneumonia Assess for ICU admission especially if CURB-65 is >4

Pneumonia is an **acute lower respiratory tract (LRT) illness**, usually due to **infection**, associated with **fever, focal chest symptoms (±signs)** and **new shadowing on chest X-ray (CXR)** (Fig. 36a). Table 1 lists microorganisms and pathological insults that cause pneumonia.

Classification

In the clinical situation, **microbiological classification** of pneumonia is not practical as causative organisms may not be identified or diagnosis takes several days. Likewise, **anatomical** (radiographical) appearance (e.g. lobar pneumonia (affecting one lobe) or bronchopneumonia (widespread, patchy involvement)) gives little practical information about cause. The following classification is widely accepted:

• **Community-acquired pneumonia (CAP):** describes LRT infections occurring within 48 hours of hospital admission in patients who have not been hospitalized for more than 14 days. The most frequently identified organism is *Streptococcus pneumoniae* (20–75%). *Mycoplasma pneumoniae*, *Chlamydia pneumoniae* and *Legionalla* spp., the 'atypical' bacterial pathogens (2–25%) and viral infections (8–12%) are relatively common causes. *Haemophilus influenzae* and *Moraxella catarrhalis* are associated with chronic obstructive pulmonary disease (COPD) exacerbations, and staphylococcal infection may follow influenza. Alcoholic, diabetic and nursing home patients are prone to staphylococcal, anaerobic and Gram-negative organisms.

• **Hospital-acquired (nosocomial) pneumonia** (Chapter 37): any LRT infections developing more than 2 days after hospital admission. Likely organisms are Gram-negative bacilli (~70%) or staphylococcus (~15%).

• **Aspiration/anaerobic pneumonia:** bacteroides and other anaerobic infections follow aspiration of oropharyngeal contents (e.g. CVA).

• **Opportunistic pneumonia** (Chapter 39): immunosuppressed patients (e.g. steroids, chemotherapy and HIV) are susceptible to viral, fungal and mycobacterial infections, in addition to other bacterial organisms.

• **Recurrent pneumonia:** due to aerobic and anaerobic organisms occurs in cystic fibrosis and bronchiectasis.

Epidemiology

Annual incidence: 5–11 cases per 1000 adult population; 15–45% require hospitalization (1–4 cases per 1000) of whom 5–10% are treated in ICU. Incidence is highest in the very young and elderly. **Mortality:** 5–12% in hospitalized patients; 25–50% in ICU patients. **Seasonal variation:** with peaks (e.g. *Mycoplasma* in autumn, *Staphylococcus* in spring) and annual cycles occur (e.g. 4-yearly *Mycoplasma* epidemics). Frequent viral infections increase CAP in winter.

Risk factors

Factors associated with increased risk of CAP are listed in Table 2. **Specific risk factors** include **age** (e.g. *Mycoplasma* in young adults), **occupation** (e.g. brucellosis in abattoir workers and Q fever in sheep workers), **environment** (e.g. psittacosis with pet birds and erlichiosis due to tick bites) or **geographical** (e.g. coccidiomycosis in southwest USA). Epidemics of *Coxiella burnetti* (Q fever) or *Legionella pneumophila* are often localized (e.g. Legionnaire's disease may involve a specific hotel due to air conditioner contamination).

Diagnosis

The aims are to establish the **diagnosis**, identify **complications**, assess **severity** and determine **classification** to aid antibiotic choice.

Clinical features

These are inaccurate without a CXR and cannot predict causative organisms (i.e. 'atypical' pathogens do not have characteristic presentations). **Symptoms** may be general (e.g. malaise, fever, rigors and myalgia) or chest-specific (e.g. dyspnoea, pleurisy, cough and haemoptysis). **Signs** include cyanosis, tachycardia and tachypnoea; with focal dullness, crepitations, bronchial breathing and pleuritic rub on chest

examination. In young or old patients and atypical pneumonias (e.g. *Mycoplasma*), **non-respiratory features** (e.g. confusion, rashes and diarrhoea) may predominate. **Complications** are shown in Fig. 36e.

Investigations

Routine blood tests: white cell count (WCC) and C-reactive protein confirm infection; haemolysis and cold agglutinins occur in approximately 50% of *Mycoplasma* infection; abnormal liver function tests suggest *Legionella* or *Mycoplasma* infection. **Blood gases:** identify respiratory failure. **Microbiology:** no microorganism is isolated in approximately 33–50% of patients due to previous antibiotic therapy or inadequate specimen collection. Blood cultures in severe CAP, and sputum, pleural fluid and bronchoalveolar lavage samples, with appropriate staining, culture and assessment of antibiotic sensitivity, may determine the pathogen and effective therapy. **Serology:** identifies *Mycoplasma* infection but long processing times limit clinical value. Rapid antigen detection tests for *Legionella* (e.g. urine) and pneumococcus (e.g. serum and pleural fluid) are more useful. **Radiology:** CXR (Fig. 36a) and CT scans aid diagnosis and detect complications.

Severity assessment

The following features are associated with increased mortality and indicate the need for monitoring in ICU: **Clinical:** age more than 60 years; respiratory rate more than 30/min; diastolic blood pressure less than 60 mmHg; new atrial fibrillation; confusion; multilobar involvement; and coexisting illness. **Laboratory:** urea more than 7 mmol/L; albumin less than 35 g/L; hypoxaemia Po_2 less than 8 kPa; leucopenia (WCC $<4 \times 10^9$/L); leucocytosis (WCC $>20 \times 10^9$/L); and bacteraemia. **Severity scoring:** CRB-65 and CURB-65 scores, allocate points for **c**onfusion; **u**rea more than 7 mmol/L; **r**espiratory rate more than 30/min; low systolic (<90 mmHg) or diastolic (<60 mmHg) **b**lood pressure and age more than **65** years, to stratify patients into mortality groups suitable for different management pathways (Fig. 36c and d).

Management

Supportive measures: include oxygen to maintain P_aO_2 of more than 8 kPa ($S_aO_2 <90\%$) and intravenous fluid ($\pm$inotrope) resuscitation to ensure haemodynamic stability. **Ventilatory support:** non-invasive (e.g. continuous positive airway pressure (CPAP)) or mechanical ventilation may be required in respiratory failure (Chapter 42). **Physiotherapy and bronchoscopy:** aid sputum clearance.

Initial antibiotic therapy: represents the 'best guess', according to pneumonia classification and likely organisms, as microbiological results are not available for 12–72 hours. Therapy is adjusted when results and antibiotic sensitivities become available. The American and British Thoracic Societies (ATS, BTS) recommend the following initial antibiotic protocols for CAP:

• **Non-hospitalized patients:** usually respond to oral therapy with amoxicillin (BTS) or an advanced macrolide (e.g. clarithromycin) or doxycycline (ATS). Patients with severe symptoms or at risk for drug-resistant *S. pneumoniae* (e.g. recent antibiotics and comorbidity) are treated with a β-lactam plus a macrolide or doxycycline, or an antipneumococcal fluoroquinolone (e.g. moxifloxacin) alone.

• **Hospitalized patients:** initial therapy must cover 'atypical' organisms and *S. pneumoniae*. An intravenous macrolide is combined with a β-lactam or an antipneumococcal fluoroquinolone (ATS/BTS) or cefuroxime (BTS). If not severe, combined ampicillin and macrolide (oral or i.v.) may be adequate (BTS). Staphylococcal infection following influenza and *H. influenzae* in COPD should be covered.

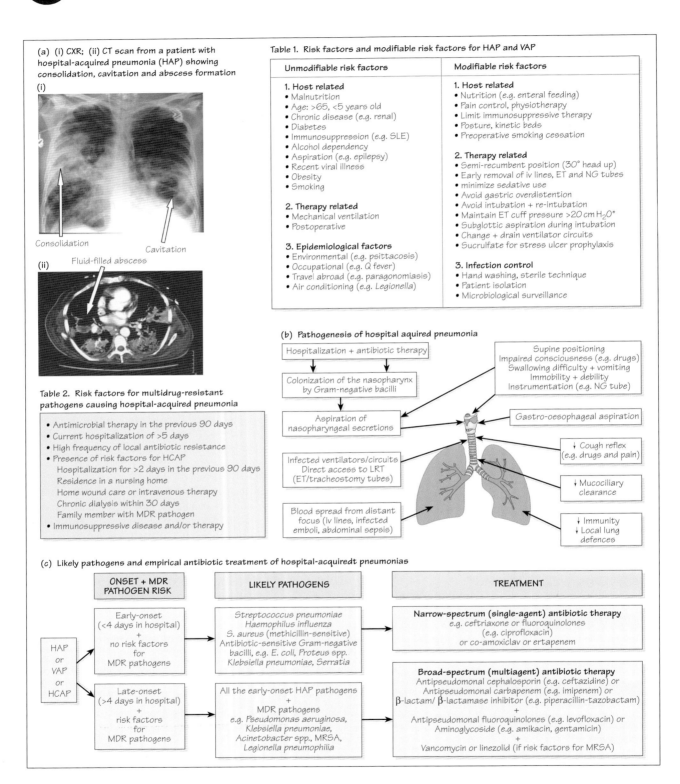

(a) (i) CXR; (ii) CT scan from a patient with hospital-acquired pneumonia (HAP) showing consolidation, cavitation and abscess formation

(i)

Consolidation   Cavitation

(ii)   Fluid-filled abscess

Table 1. Risk factors and modifiable risk factors for HAP and VAP

Unmodifiable risk factors	Modifiable risk factors
1. Host related • Malnutrition • Age: >65, <5 years old • Chronic disease (e.g. renal) • Diabetes • Immunosuppression (e.g. SLE) • Alcohol dependency • Aspiration (e.g. epilepsy) • Recent viral illness • Obesity • Smoking **2. Therapy related** • Mechanical ventilation • Postoperative **3. Epidemiological factors** • Environmental (e.g. psittacosis) • Occupational (e.g. Q fever) • Travel abroad (e.g. paragonomiasis) • Air conditioning (e.g. Legionella)	**1. Host related** • Nutrition (e.g. enteral feeding) • Pain control, physiotherapy • Limit immunosuppressive therapy • Posture, kinetic beds • Preoperative smoking cessation **2. Therapy related** • Semi-recumbent position (30° head up) • Early removal of iv lines, ET and NG tubes • minimize sedative use • Avoid gastric overdistention • Avoid intubation + re-intubation • Maintain ET cuff pressure >20 cm H_2O* • Subglottic aspiration during intubation • Change + drain ventilator circuits • Sucrulfate for stress ulcer prophylaxis **3. Infection control** • Hand washing, sterile technique • Patient isolation • Microbiological surveillance

Table 2. Risk factors for multidrug-resistant pathogens causing hospital-acquired pneumonia

• Antimicrobial therapy in the previous 90 days
• Current hospitalization of >5 days
• High frequency of local antibiotic resistance
• Presence of risk factors for HCAP
   Hospitalization for >2 days in the previous 90 days
   Residence in a nursing home
   Home wound care or intravenous therapy
   Chronic dialysis within 30 days
   Family member with MDR pathogen
• Immunosuppressive disease and/or therapy

(b) Pathogenesis of hospital aquired pneumonia

Hospitalization + antibiotic therapy

Colonization of the nasopharynx by Gram-negative bacilli

Aspiration of nasopharyngeal secretions

Infected ventilators/circuits Direct access to LRT (ET/tracheostomy tubes)

Blood spread from distant focus (iv lines, infected emboli, abdominal sepsis)

Supine positioning
Impaired consciousness (e.g. drugs)
Swallowing difficulty + vomiting
Immobility + debility
Instrumentation (e.g. NG tube)

Gastro-oesophageal aspiration

↓ Cough reflex (e.g. drugs and pain)

↓ Mucociliary clearance

↓ Immunity
↓ Local lung defences

(c) Likely pathogens and empirical antibiotic treatment of hospital-acquiredt pneumonias

ONSET + MDR PATHOGEN RISK	LIKELY PATHOGENS	TREATMENT
HAP or VAP or HCAP → Early-onset (<4 days in hospital) + no risk factors for MDR pathogens	*Streptococcus pneumoniae* *Haemophilus influenza* *S. aureus* (methicillin-sensitive) Antibiotic-sensitive Gram-negative bacilli, e.g. *E. coli, Proteus spp.* *Klebsiella pneumoniae, Serratia*	**Narrow-spectrum (single-agent) antibiotic therapy** e.g. ceftriaxone or fluoroquinolones (e.g. ciprofloxacin) or co-amoxiclav or ertapenem
Late-onset (>4 days in hospital) + risk factors for MDR pathogens	All the early-onset HAP pathogens + MDR pathogens e.g. *Pseudomonas aeruginosa,* *Klebsiella pneumoniae,* *Acinetobacter spp.,* MRSA, *Legionella pneumophilia*	**Broad-spectrum (multiagent) antibiotic therapy** Antipseudomonal cephalosporin (e.g. ceftazidine) or Antipseudomonal carbapenem (e.g. imipenem) or β-lactam/ β-lactamase inhibitor (e.g. piperacillin-tazobactam) + Antipseudomonal fluoroquinolones (e.g. levofloxacin) or Aminoglycoside (e.g. amikacin, gentamicin) + Vancomycin or linezolid (if risk factors for MRSA)

Hospital-acquired (nosocomial) pneumonia (HAP) including ventilator-associated pneumonia (VAP) and healthcare-associated pneumonia (HCAP) affects 0.5–2% of hospital patients and is a leading cause of nosocomial infection (i.e. with wound, urinary tract and bloodstream). Pathogenesis, causative organisms and outcome differ from community-acquired pneumonia (CAP). Preventative measures and early antibiotic therapy, guided by awareness of the role of multidrug-resistant (MDR) pathogens, improve outcome.

Definitions

HAP: pulmonary infection developing more than 48 hours after hospital admission that was not incubating at the time of admission. **VAP:** pneumonia developing more than 48–72 hours after endotracheal intubation. **HCAP:** includes any patient admitted to hospital for more than 2 days within 90 days of the infection, residing in a nursing home, receiving therapy (e.g. wound care and intravenous therapy) within 30 days of the current infection, or attending a hospital or haemodialysis clinic.

Epidemiology

Incidence: varies between 5 and 10 episodes per 1000 discharges and is highest on surgical and ICU wards and in teaching hospitals. It lengthens hospital stay by between 3 and 14 days per patient. The risk of HAP increases 6- to 20-fold during mechanical ventilation (MV), and in ICU, it accounts for 25% of infections and approximately 50% of prescribed antibiotics. VAP accounts for more than 80% of all HAP and occurs in 9–27% of intubated patients. **Risk factors:** include those that predispose to CAP and factors associated with HAP pathogenesis, some of which can be **prevented** (Table 1). **Mortality:** between 30 and 70%. **Early-onset HAP/VAP** (<4 days in hospital) is usually caused by antibiotic-sensitive bacteria and carries a better prognosis than **late-onset HAP/VAP** (>4 days in hospital), which is associated with MDR pathogens. In early-onset HAP/VAP, prior antibiotic therapy or hospitalization predisposes to MDR pathogens and is treated as late-onset HAP/VAP. Bacteraemia, medical rather than surgical illness, VAP and late or ineffective antibiotic therapy also increase mortality.

Pathogenesis

Oropharyneal colonization with enteric Gram-negative bacteria occurs in most hospital patients due to immobility, impaired consciousness, instrumentation (e.g. nasogastric tubes), poor hygiene or inhibition of gastric acid secretion. Subsequent aspiration of nasopharyngeal secretions (±gastric contents) causes HAP (Fig. 37b).

Aetiology

Time of onset (early/late) and risk factors for infection with MDR organisms (Table 2) determine potential pathogens (Fig. 37c). Aerobic Gram-negative bacilli (e.g. *Klebsiella pneumoniae*, *Pseudomonas aeruginosa*, *Escherichia coli*) cause approximately 60–70% of infections and *Staphylococcus aureus* approximately 10–15%. *Streptococcus pneumoniae* and *Haemophilus influenza* may be isolated in early-onset HAP/VAP. In ICU, more than 50% of *S. aureus* infections are methicillin-resistant (MRSA). *S. aureus* is more common in diabetics and ICU patients.

Diagnosis

Requires both *clinical* and *microbiological* assessment. It may be difficult as (i) clinical features are non-specific or confused with concurrent illness (e.g. acute respiratory distress syndrome (ARDS)); and (ii) previous antibiotics limit microbiological evaluation. **Clinical:** HAP is suspected when new radiographical infiltrates occur with features suggestive of infection (e.g. fever >38°C, purulent sputum, leucocytosis and hypoxaemia). **Diagnostic tests:** confirm infection and determine the causative organism (±antibiotic sensitivity). They include routine blood counts, blood gases, serology, blood cultures, pleural effusions aspiration, sputum, endotracheal aspirate and bronchoalveolar lavage microbiology and CXR. CT scanning (Fig. 37a) aids diagnosis and detects **complications** (e.g. abscesses).

Management

Early diagnosis and treatment improves morbidity and mortality and requires constant vigilance in hospital patients. Antibiotic therapy must not be delayed while awaiting microbiological results.

Supportive therapy

This includes supplemental **oxygen** to maintain P_aO_2 of more than 8 kPa (S_aO_2 <90%), **intravenous fluids (±vasopressors/inotropes)** for haemodynamic stability and **ventilatory support** (e.g. continuous positive airway pressure (CPAP), MV) in respiratory failure. **Physiotherapy** and **analgesia** aid sputum clearance postoperatively and in the immobilized patient. **Semi-recumbent** (i.e. 30° bed-head elevation) nursing of bed-bound patients reduces aspiration risk. Strict glycaemic control and attention to other modifiable risk factors (Table 1) may improve outcome.

Antibiotic therapy

This is empirical while awaiting microbiological guidance. The key decision is whether the patient has risk factors for MDR organisms. Figure 37c illustrates the American Thoracic Society (ATS) guidelines for initial, intravenous antibiotic therapy. Local patterns of antibiotic resistance are used to modify these protocols.

• In **early-onset HAP/VAP** with no risk factors for MDR organisms, **monotherapy** with a β-lactam/β-lactamase, third-generation cephalosporin or fluoroquinolone antibiotic is advised.

• In **late-onset HAP/VAP** with risk factors for MDR pathogens (Table 2), **combination therapy** with broad-spectrum antibiotics to cover MDR Gram-negative bacilli and MRSA (e.g. vancomycin) is required (Fig. 37c). Adjunctive therapy with inhaled aminoglycosides or polymyxin is considered in patients not improving with systemic therapy.

A short course of therapy (e.g. 7 days) is appropriate if the clinical response is good. Aggressive or resistant pathogens (e.g. *P. aeruginosa*, *S. aureus*) may require 14–21 days' treatment. Therapy is focused on causative organisms when culture data are available and unnecessary antibiotics are withdrawn. Sterile cultures (in the absence of new antibiotics for >72 hours) virtually rules out HAP.

Other pneumonias

Aspiration/anaerobic pneumonia: *Bacteroides* and other anaerobic infections follow aspiration of oropharyngeal contents due to laryngeal incompetence or reduced consciousness (e.g. cerebrovascular accident; CVA, drugs). Lung abscesses are common. Antibiotic therapy should include anaerobic coverage (e.g. metronidazole).

Pneumonia during immunosuppression (Chapter 39): HIV, transplant and chemotherapy patients are susceptible to viral (e.g. cytomegalovirus), fungal (e.g. *Aspergillus*) and mycobacterial infections, in addition to the normal range of organisms. HIV patients with CD4 counts of less than 200/mm^3 also develop opportunistic infections such as *Pneumocystis carinii* pneumonia (PCP) or toxoplasma. Severely immunocompromised patients require broad-spectrum antibiotic, antifungal and antiviral regimens. PCP is treated with steroids and high-dose co-trimoxazole.

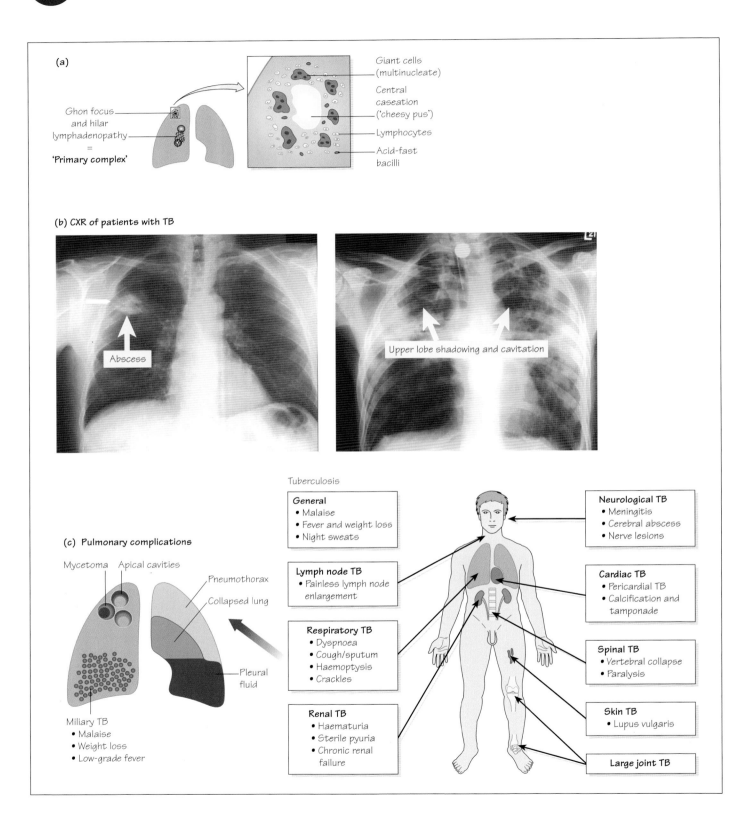

(a)

Ghon focus and hilar lymphadenopathy = 'Primary complex'

Giant cells (multinucleate)

Central caseation ('cheesy pus')

Lymphocytes

Acid-fast bacilli

(b) CXR of patients with TB

Abscess

Upper lobe shadowing and cavitation

Tuberculosis

General
• Malaise
• Fever and weight loss
• Night sweats

Lymph node TB
• Painless lymph node enlargement

Respiratory TB
• Dyspnoea
• Cough/sputum
• Haemoptysis
• Crackles

Renal TB
• Haematuria
• Sterile pyuria
• Chronic renal failure

Neurological TB
• Meningitis
• Cerebral abscess
• Nerve lesions

Cardiac TB
• Pericardial TB
• Calcification and tamponade

Spinal TB
• Vertebral collapse
• Paralysis

Skin TB
• Lupus vulgaris

Large joint TB

(c) Pulmonary complications

Mycetoma   Apical cavities

Pneumothorax

Collapsed lung

Pleural fluid

Miliary TB
• Malaise
• Weight loss
• Low-grade fever

Worldwide, tuberculosis (TB) affects 10 million people and causes 2 million deaths each year. In developed countries it is uncommon, affecting approximately 1 per 10000 population. Pulmonary TB is most common in Asian, Chinese and West Indian people. Airborne transmission and close contact spread the disease. Those who are elderly, malnourished or immunosuppressed (HIV infection, diabetes mellitus, corticosteroid therapy, alcoholism, intercurrent lymphoma) are more susceptible. Improved housing and nutrition reduce incidence.

Pathogenesis

Primary pulmonary TB is caused by the acid-fast bacillus *Mycobacterium tuberculosis*. The inhaled bacillus infects well-ventilated, poorly perfused upper lung lobes subpleurally. A **granuloma** forms (Fig. 38a) known as the **Ghon focus**, and with the enlarged hilar lymph node draining the affected lung is known as the '**primary complex**' (Fig. 38a). This occurs over 3–8 weeks, and is accompanied by development of an inflammatory reaction to injection of tubercular protein (**tuberculin**) into the skin, which can be used as a diagnostic test (**Mantoux** or **Heaf** test). Complete healing usually follows, with fibrosis and calcification of the Ghon focus and immunity to further infection.

Post-primary pulmonary TB occurs if the Ghon focus fails to heal due to poor host defences, or following reactivation. It is potentially fatal. Local dissemination causes **tuberculous pneumonia** and **pleural effusions**. Bloodborne spread may affect the meninges or individual organs. In a few cases, widespread infection involves many tissues (**miliary TB**).

Clinical features

Primary pulmonary TB usually occurs at an early age. Often asymptomatic with no clinical signs, it may cause a mild febrile illness, **erythema nodosum** (painful, indurated shin lesions) and small pleural effusions. Bronchial compression by lymphadenopathy may cause wheeze and occasionally lobar collapse followed by late **bronchiectasis** (Chapter 34).

Post-primary TB develops over months, with malaise, anorexia, weight loss, night sweats and a productive cough. Breathlessness, chest pain, haemoptysis and cervical lymphadenopathy may occur. Clinical signs of pneumonia and pleural effusion are common, whereas lupus vulgaris (an indolent skin infection) is less frequent. **Miliary TB** presents with a non-specific pyrexial illness, malaise and weight loss. Sparse clinical signs include hepatomegaly and choroidal tubercles in the retina.

Investigation

Blood tests may detect anaemia, decreased sodium and increased calcium.

Mantoux test: strongly positive in post-primary pulmonary TB (>5 mm skin induration with 10 units of intradermal tuberculin; read at 3 days). Often negative in miliary TB (reduced host response) and HIV (reduced cellular immunity).

Heaf test (screening test; now less commonly used): a ring of six pinpricks is made through a tuberculin solution on the forearm. No response at 4–7 days (grade 0) demonstrates lack of immunity; 4–6 discrete nodules (grade 1) or a ring formed by coalition of all pinpricks (grade 2) indicates immunity. A single nodule formed by infilling of the ring (grade 3) represents recent contact or early tuberculous infection, and a nodule of more than 5–7 mm with surface vesicles or ulceration (grade 4) suggests infection.

Microbiology: the acid-fast bacilli may be detected in sputum or lung washings using Ziehl–Neelsen stain. However, bacilli are slow growing, and culture and drug sensitivities take 4–6 weeks. Bone marrow or cerebrospinal fluid (CSF) culture may confirm the diagnosis of miliary TB.

Histopathology: pleural aspiration with biopsy confirms TB in approximately 90% of patients with pleural effusions. Liver biopsy will isolate miliary TB in approximately 60% of cases.

Chest radiography (Fig. 38b): upper lobe shadowing is suggestive. Apical cavities, pleural effusions and pneumothoraxes may occur. In miliary TB, widespread small nodules (2–3 mm diameter) are diffusely spread throughout the lungs (miliary shadowing), and are easily missed.

Drug therapy

Prognosis is good if the patient is not immunocompromised. Good nutrition, reduced alcohol consumption and **compliance with drug therapy** are important factors. Uncomplicated pulmonary TB is treated for 6 months. Initially, at least three drugs are used to prevent development of resistant strains. The recommended regimen is rifampicin, pyrazinamide and isoniazid for 2 months, followed by rifampicin and isoniazid for 4 months. Additional pyridoxine prevents isoniazid-induced peripheral neuropathy. Liver function should be monitored, as rifampicin and pyrazinamide can cause liver dysfunction. If drug resistance is suspected (TB recurrence in a non-compliant patient) then a four-drug regimen (adding ethambutol) may be initiated. When culture results are available, alternative drugs replace those to which the mycobacterium is not sensitive. Ethambutol (monitor colour vision for optic neuritis), streptomycin (monitor plasma levels to avoid hearing impairment) or ciprofloxacin may be used. In severe pulmonary TB, corticosteroids occasionally improve results.

In some organs (e.g. bone), TB is treated for longer, often with additional drugs. In meningeal or cerebral TB, a four-drug regimen for 12 months with additional steroids is recommended, to ensure adequate brain penetration and to prevent cranial nerve compression by meningeal scarring.

Complications

Reactivation of old tuberculous scars may occur when a patient is immunocompromised (Fig. 38c). Chemoprophylaxis with isoniazid is often given before immunosuppressive treatment (chemotherapy, organ transplantation). Bronchiectasis and lung cavities with secondary fungal infections (mycetoma), cranial nerve lesions and renal tract obstructions may develop due to scarring associated with healing after TB. Non-compliance or inadequate treatment results in multiresistant strains of mycobacteria that may be very difficult to eradicate. Compulsory supervision and isolation of these patients may be required.

Prevention and contact tracing

Vaccination of non-immune subjects with **BCG** (bacille Calmette–Guérin), a non-virulent strain of bovine TB, produces immunity and reduces the risk of pulmonary TB by 70%. Community health services **must be notified** when a patient is diagnosed with TB, to trace contacts and prevent spread. Contacts are screened with a Mantoux test. If this suggests a risk of infection, then chest radiography and appropriate follow-up are arranged.

(a) Causes of new pulmonary infiltrates

Infectious
- Bacterial pneumonia
- Fungal pneumonia (e.g. aspergillosis)
- Opportunistic pneumonia (e.g. PCP)
- Viral pneumonoia

Non-infectious
- Pulmonary oedema, ARDS
- Radiation pneumonitis
- Drug-induced, e.g. amiodarone, busulphan
- Malignant infiltration
- Pulmonary haemorrhage
- Non-specific interstitial pneumonitis

(b) Infectious causes of respiratory disease in immunocompromised patients

Immunological defect	Clinical conditions	Types of infection
Neutropaenia	Chemotherapy, leukaemia, aplastic anaemia	Bacterial (e.g. E. coli, staph aureus) Fungal (e.g. aspergillus)
Impaired T-cell function	Transplantation, steroids, lymphoma, HIV infection, chemotherapy	Bacteria (e.g. mycobacteria), fungi (e.g. PCP), viruses (e.g. CMV)
Impaired B-cell function	Lymphoma, leukaemia, myeloma, hypogammaglobulinaemia	Streptococcus pneumoniae, Haemophilus influenza
Impaired compliment	Mannose lectin deficiency, complement deficiency	Streptococcus pneumonia

(c) Clinical features of AIDS
Causes of respiratory disease and CXR infiltrates in HIV-infected patients

Clinical features and diseases that are indicators of AIDS

Cerebral
HIV encephalopathy, dementia
Cerebral toxoplasmosis
Cryptococcus neoformans
Primary brain lymphoma

Respiratory
Pneumocystis pneumonia
Mycobacterium avium complex
Mycobacterium tuberculosis
Pneumonia (e.g. S. pneumoniae)

General
Weight loss, fatigue
Lymphadenopathy
CMV retinitis

Gastrointestinal
Diarrhoea
Cytomegalovirus colitis
Oral + oesophageal candida
Small bowel lymphoma

Skin
Herpes simplex
Kaposi's sarcoma
Dermatitis

Malignancy
Non-Hodgkins lymphoma
Burkitts lymphoma

Blood
Lymphopaenia
Bacteraemia

Causes of chest disease + CXR infiltrates in HIV-infected patients (*commonest)

Infection*
- Bacterial (e.g. S. Pneumoniae)
- Pneumocystis pneumonia
- Fungal (e.g. cryptococcus)
- Mycobacterial infection (e.g. MTB, MAC)
- Viral (e.g CMV)

Malignancy
Non-Hodgkin lymphoma
Kaposi's sarcoma
Burkitt's lymphoma
Lung cancer

Drug toxicity
e.g. amiodarone, busulphan

Interstitial pneumonitis
e.g. Non-specific interstitial pneumonitis
Lymphocytic interstital pneumonitis

General causes
Heart failure, pulmonary oedema
Sepsis-induced acute respiratory distress syndrome (ARDS)
Radiation pneumonitis
Pulmonary haemorrhage

(d) Pneumocystis Jirovecii pneumonia (PCP) showing bilateral diffuse infiltrates

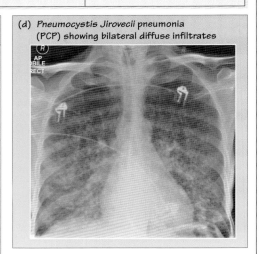

(e) Cerebral toxoplasmosis with ring enhancement on a post-contrast CT brain scan

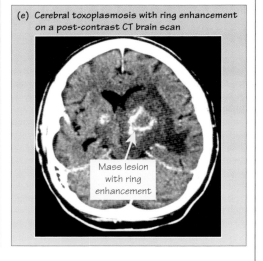

Mass lesion with ring enhancement

The immune system is most frequently impaired after chemotherapy and in patients with human immunodeficiency virus (HIV) infection. Immunodeficiency also occurs in patients with malignancies of the lymphoproliferative system (e.g. leukaemia), immediately following bone marrow transplants (BMT) and in those on immunosuppressive drugs (e.g. steroids and azothioprine) particularly after transplant surgery (e.g. renal). Malnutrition or chronic illness (e.g. diabetes) may also impair immunity. Respiratory disease is particularly common in the immunocompromised host.

Clinical presentation is often non-specific (i.e. fever, dyspnoea, hypoxia, cough and chest discomfort) and investigation inconclusive making diagnosis difficult. In particular, pulmonary infiltrates are not always due to infection (Fig. 39a). Clinical clues include rate of onset (i.e. rapid in bacterial infection and slow with malignancy), drug therapy (e.g. methotrexate) and extrapulmonary features (e.g. Kaposi's sarcoma). Establishing the diagnosis may require invasive techniques (e.g. biopsy) with associated risks (e.g. haemorrhage).

Investigations include blood and pleural fluid microscopy, culture and serology. Sputum for *Aspergillus* or mycobacteria and 'induced' sputum for *Pneumocystis jiroveci* pneumoniae (PCP). CXR findings may be non-specific (e.g. diffuse infiltrates). Chest CT scans assess extent of lung involvement, aid invasive sampling and may be diagnostic (e.g. halo sign of aspergillosis). Consider early bronchoalveolar lavage (BAL) with microbiology, stains (e.g. fungus and virus), immunofluorescence (e.g. PCP) and serology (e.g. CMV and *Cryptococcus*) as this is often diagnostic (50–60%). Transbronchial, fine-needle and surgical lung biopsies have risks but may aid diagnosis.

Diagnosis is due to respiratory infection in more than 75% of cases:
• **Infection** depends on the immunological defect (Fig. 39b) and prophylactic therapy (e.g. septrin for PCP).
• **Non-infectious causes** present with similar clinical and CXR features to infection and include pulmonary oedema, ARDS, malignancy (e.g. lymphoma), diffuse alveolar haemorrhage, pulmonary embolism, drug-induced disease (e.g. methotrexate), BMT-associated idiopathic pneumonia, radiation pneumonitis and chronic graft-versus-host disease. More than one cause is often present (30%).

Treatment is often empirical as antibiotic therapy cannot be delayed in febrile neutropaenic patients, in whom infection is a medical emergency. Blood cultures should always precede antibiotics.
• **Antibiotic** choice depends on the clinical situation and local antibiotic policy. Initial treatment of immunosuppressed cases involves broad-spectrum antibiotics (±antiviral and antifungal agents). Treatment should be adjusted when results are available. PCP and CMV therapy have significant toxic side effects, but if suspicion is high, treatment is started empirically. PCP can be diagnosed for up to 2 weeks after onset of therapy. Treatment of mycobacteria is only started after definitive diagnosis.
• **Steroid therapy** is recommended in PCP, radiation/drug-induced pneumonitis, BMT idiopathic pneumonia and alveolar haemorrhage.
• **Supportive therapy** includes supplemental oxygen and ventilatory support. Respiratory failure has a poor outcome in these patients.

Respiratory manifestations in the HIV-positive patient (Fig. 39c)

Acquired immune deficiency syndrome (AIDS) is due to infection with HIV, which impairs and depletes CD4 T-lymphocytes (Chapter 18). Reduction in T-lymphocyte availability predisposes to viral or fungal infections and neoplasia (Fig. 39e). Highly active antiretroviral therapy (HAART) allows T-lymphocyte population recovery, reduces susceptibility to infection and improves survival. Nevertheless, HIV patients are at increased risk of infection with common bacteria, PCP, mycobacteria and fungi. Factors determining the type and risk of infection include the use of prophylactic antibiotics (e.g. PCP prophylaxis), source of infection (e.g. TB is more common with drug abuse) and geography (e.g. histoplasmosis and coccidioidomycosis are more common in the USA). Extrapulmonary features (e.g. Kaposi's sarcoma) may suggest the cause of pulmonary disease.

1 Infectious causes
• **Bacterial pneumonia** (e.g. *Streptococcus pneumoniae*, *Staphylococcus aureus* and *Nocardia*) is the commonest chest infection in HIV patients. Rapid onset of high fever, purulent sputum and pleuritic chest pain help distinguish bacterial pneumonia from PCP. *Legionella* infections are more common in HIV patients.
• ***Pneumocystis jirovecii* pneumonia** occurs in severely immunocompromised patients (CD4 $<200 \times 10^6$/L). It has been less common since the use of septrin prophylaxis in high-risk cases. It presents with gradual onset of fever, dry cough, exertional dyspnoea, chest tightness, tachypnoea and rarely pneumothorax. Exercise-induced desaturation progresses to resting hypoxaemia. CXR shows bilateral alveolar infiltrates (Fig. 39d) but may be normal (10%) or show focal consolidation. Diagnosis requires detection of pneumocysts in induced sputum (~60–70%) or BAL (>90%). High-dose co-trimoxazole is the most effective therapy but may cause rashes (~30%), vomiting and blood disorders. Pentamidine and dapsone are second-line alternatives. High-dose steroids reduce alveolitis, respiratory failure and mortality.
• **Mycobacteria** (e.g. *Mycobacterium tuberculosis* (MTB), *Mycobacterium avium* complex (MAC)). Globally 10% of MTB cases are also infected with HIV. However, co-infection rates vary geographically affecting 35–40% in sub-Saharan cases and 2.7% in the UK. HIV patients with previous MTB exposure have a 10% chance of reactivation, and approximately 33% of patients exposed to MTB develop primary disease. Advanced immunosuppression is typically associated with diffuse pulmonary involvement, mediastinal adenopathy and extrapulmonary involvement. Symptoms may deteriorate with the onset of HAART due to immune reconstitution. Non-tuberculous mycobacterial (NTM) infection is due to MAC in more than 90% of cases. MAC treatment is lifelong unless immune restoration is achieved with HARRT.
• **Viral** (e.g. influenza and herpes simplex). *Cytomegalovirus* (CMV) is ubiquitous and normally harmless but can cause life-threatening pneumonia in the immunocompromised. Diagnosis requires evidence of viraemia (i.e. antigen/PCR testing on blood/BAL) or tissue invasion (e.g. 'owl eye' inclusion bodies in infected biopsy cells). Ganciclovir is the most effective antiviral agent.
• **Fungal** (e.g. *Aspergillus*). *Cryptococcus neoformans* propagates asymptomatically in alveoli following inhalation (from bird droppings), before migrating to the CNS where it causes meningitis (±encephalitis). Onset is acute or chronic with fever, cough and non-specific CXR changes. The cryptococcal antigen test and India ink stain establish the diagnosis. Treatment is with amphotericin, flucytosine and fluconazole. In endemic areas, **histoplasmosis** and **coccidioidomycosis** may cause respiratory disease.

2 Non-infectious causes
• **Malignancies** are occasionally confused with infection in HIV patients. **Kaposi's sarcoma** is a tumour of vascular origin associated with human herpesvirus 8 infection. Clinical manifestations range from asymptomatic incidental discovery to fulminating disease, causing respiratory failure. **Non-Hodgkin's lymphoma** occurs in advanced immunosuppression and is typically aggressive B-cell or Burkitt's lymphoma, suggesting pre-existing herpesvirus infection. **Lung cancer** is also increased in HIV patients.
• **Interstitial pneumonitis** (e.g. NSIP, LIP, Chapter 30).
• **Drug-induced** lung disease or **heart failure**.

40 Lung cancer

(a) Mass on CT: a >3 cm spiculated mass is seen in upper lobe of the right lung

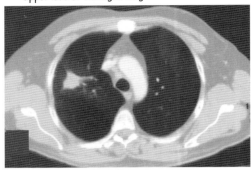

(b) Fibreoptic bronchoscopy showing tumour invading bronchus

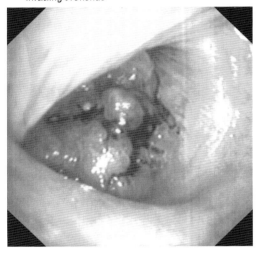

(c) CXR showing squamous cell tumour in hilar region

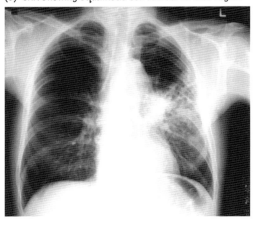

(d) Staging system for non-small cell lung cancers

Stage	T (tumour)	N (node)	M (metastasis)	Key
IA	T1	N0	M0	**T1:** ≤3 cm without division
IB	T2	N0	M0	**T2:** >3 cm, or invasion of main bronchus
IIA	T1	N1	M0	>2 cm from main carina, or invades
IIB	T2	N1	M0	visceral pleura, or bronchus causing
	T3	N0	M0	obstruction
				T3: Invades chest wall or pleura, or main bronchus <2 cm from main carina
				T4: Invades adjacent structure, malignant effusion, satellite nodules
IIIA	T1, 2, 3	N2	M0	**N0:** No lymph node metastasis
	T3	N1	M0	**N1:** Ipsilateral hilar lymph nodes
IIIB	T1, 2, 3, 4	N3	M0	**N2:** Ipsilateral mediastinal or subcarinal lymph nodes
	T4	N1, 2	M0	**N3:** Contralateral, scalene or supraclavicular lymph nodes
IV	T1–4	N0–3	M1	**M0:** No distant metastasis
				M1: Any distant metastasis

(e) Survival for non-small cell cancer

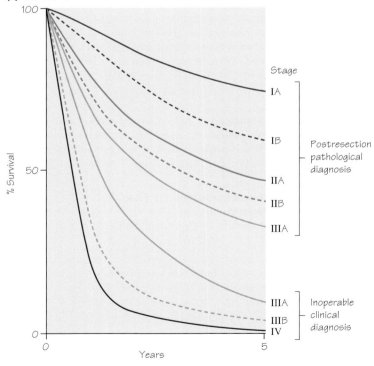

 The Respiratory System at a Glance, 3e. By J.P.T. Ward, J. Ward, R.M. Leach. Published 2010 Blackwell Publishing Ltd.

More people die in the USA and Europe from **lung cancer** than from breast, prostate and colon cancer combined. Furthermore, the number of cases is likely to increase in the next 25 years due to continued use of cigarettes, particularly in women. Lung cancer has a **worse prognosis** than other common cancers, with an overall **5-year survival** of **13%**.

Risks

Cigarette smoking accounts for the vast majority of lung cancer cases. Risk is directly related to the duration and number of cigarettes smoked, age of initiation, depth of inhalation and levels of tar and nicotine. In heavy smokers (>20 packs/years) the lifetime risk of lung cancer is 10%, 10–30 times greater than for lifelong non-smokers (<0.3%). After quitting cigarettes, risk gradually declines over 15 years, but remains 2–5 times greater than in non-smokers. **Passive smoking** in non-smokers may increase the risk by approximately 1.5%.

Asbestos exposure is the most common occupational risk for lung cancer (Chapter 33). Tobacco smoke is synergistic with asbestosis, increasing the relative risk to 6–60 times that of a non-smoker. **Radon gas**, found naturally in rocks, soil and ground water, may also increase risk.

Classification

Lung cancers are divided pathologically into **small cell** (**SC**, 20–30% of total) and **non-small cell** (**NSC**, 70–80% of total) types. **NSC** types are grouped due to their similar biology, treatment and prognosis, and include **squamous cells** (30%), **large cells** (15%) and **adenocarcinoma** (33%), which are increasing in prevalence, especially in women. **Adenocarcinomas** typically present as a peripheral nodule (<3 cm) or mass (>3 cm); they are the most common type in non-smokers, and mainly arise in areas of pulmonary scarring. Bronchoalveolar cell carcinoma is an adenocarcinoma variant with low metastatic potential. **Squamous cell carcinomas** arise from the bronchial epithelium, and generally present as a central mass with tumour visible in the airway (Fig. 40a and b), often with symptoms due to local tumour invasion (cough, haemoptysis, chest pain and hoarseness). **Large cell carcinoma** is undifferentiated, and lacks the histological features of adenocarcinoma or squamous cell carcinoma; it generally presents as a large peripheral mass, often with metastases. **SC** carcinomas arise from neuroendocrine cells in the bronchial submucosa, and typically present as a central mass with lymph node enlargement. These are aggressive tumours that invade lymphatics and blood vessels. Nearly all have metastasized at diagnosis.

Presentation

Less than 10% of lung cancers are discovered incidentally in asymptomatic patients. Most patients are 50–70 years of age, with non-specific symptoms including new unresolving cough, haemoptysis, chest pain, hoarseness, dyspnoea on exertion, malaise and weight loss. Symptoms due to haematogenous **extrathoracic metastasis** to bone, liver, bone marrow, adrenals and brain are present in around one-third of patients at diagnosis.

Paraneoplastic syndromes – signs or symptoms associated with lung cancers that are not related directly to metastatic tumour – may precede radiographical demonstration. They may be due to secretion of hormones or hormone-like substances from tumours, or serum **autoantibodies** (e.g. anti-Hu) related to tumour antigens. SC carcinoma is associated with most paraneoplastic syndromes including Cushing's syndrome, syndrome of inappropriate secretion of antidiuretic hormone (SIADH), Lambert–Eaton syndrome, cerebellar ataxia or idiopathic orthostatic hypotension. Squamous cell cancer may cause hypercalcaemia from release of parathyroid hormone-related peptide.

Physical findings in the lung are related to disease extent. Small **parenchymal nodules** are undetectable by physical examination. Focal findings may be due to atelectasis, airway invasion, pleural effusion (Chapter 32) or supraclavicular adenopathy. Invasion of adjacent structures may cause superior vena cava syndrome (obstruction), Horner's syndrome (autonomic overactivity) or brachial plexopathy. Digital clubbing or hypertrophic pulmonary osteoarthropathy may be present.

Evaluation

Evaluation of patients with suspected lung cancer should include demonstration of **malignancy**, **staging** and **suitability for therapy**. Radiographs provide information regarding the size and location of the tumour, benign calcification, involvement of adjacent structures, atelectasis, pleural effusion and adenopathy (Fig. 40c). **Computed tomography** (**CT**) **scans** are superior to plain X-rays. If a focal lesion does not change in 2 years, it is unlikely to be malignant. **Positron emission tomography** (**PET**) **scanning** has a high sensitivity for distinguishing benign from malignant nodules and for detecting nodal or distant metastases.

Staging is assessment of the extent of the tumour, and largely determines treatment options and prognosis. Separate staging systems are used for SC and NSC cancers. **SC cancer** is staged as either **limited** or **extensive** disease. **Limited disease** describes tumour confined to one hemithorax, including malignant pleural effusion and supraclavicular lymph node metastasis. **Extensive disease** describes metastatic spread beyond the hemithorax. SC cancer is generally an incurable disease. Standard therapy for limited disease (33%) is combination of chemotherapy and radiotherapy, with response rates approaching 90%; median survival with therapy is approximately 18 months. Standard therapy for extensive disease (66%) is chemotherapy. The response rate is approximately 70%, treatment prolonging median survival from approximately 3 months to approximately 1 year.

NSC cancer staging is based on the **tumour** (T), **node** (N) and **metastasis** (M) classification system (Fig. 40d). **T3** tumours invade thoracic structures that are potentially resectable, and **T4** tumours include malignant effusions or tumours invading non-resectable structures. Summation of **TNM categories** determines the stage of disease and treatment, and predicts survival (Fig. 40e). In functional patients with **stage I** or **II** disease and adequate pulmonary reserve (postoperative FEV_1 >800 mL), **surgical resection** is optimal. Some patients with **stage IIIA** disease are surgical candidates. Patients with **stage IIIB** or **IV** disease are not candidates for curative resection. Unresectable disease is generally treated with **chemotherapy** and **radiation therapy**, or radiation alone. **Stage IV** disease is incurable (median survival 6–12 months). Treatment options are palliative. Painful bone metastases, brain metastasis or airway obstruction may improve with directed therapy. The benefit of aggressive chemotherapy for patients with advanced disease is modest. **Platinum** and **taxol-based** chemotherapy regimens are currently most common for NSC cancer.

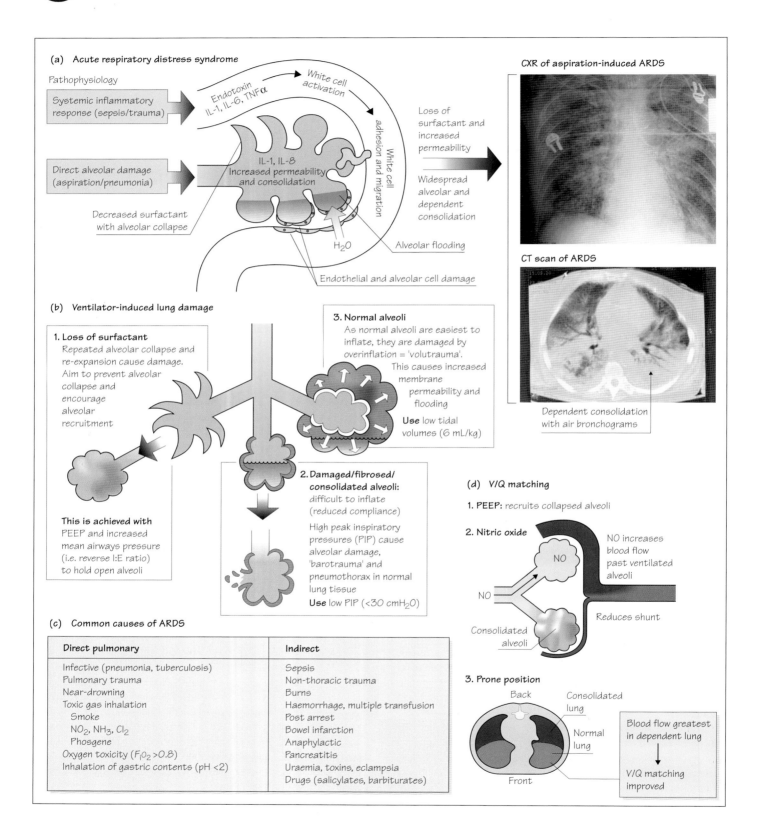

(a) Acute respiratory distress syndrome

Pathophysiology

Systemic inflammatory response (sepsis/trauma)

Endotoxin IL-1, IL-6, TNFα

White cell activation

White cell adhesion and migration

IL-1, IL-8 Increased permeability and consolidation

Direct alveolar damage (aspiration/pneumonia)

Decreased surfactant with alveolar collapse

H_2O

Loss of surfactant and increased permeability

Widespread alveolar and dependent consolidation

Alveolar flooding

Endothelial and alveolar cell damage

CXR of aspiration-induced ARDS

CT scan of ARDS

Dependent consolidation with air bronchograms

(b) Ventilator-induced lung damage

1. Loss of surfactant
Repeated alveolar collapse and re-expansion cause damage. Aim to prevent alveolar collapse and encourage alveolar recruitment

This is achieved with
PEEP and increased mean airways pressure (i.e. reverse I:E ratio) to hold open alveoli

3. Normal alveoli
As normal alveoli are easiest to inflate, they are damaged by overinflation = 'volutrauma'. This causes increased membrane permeability and flooding
Use low tidal volumes (6 mL/kg)

2. Damaged/fibrosed/ consolidated alveoli:
difficult to inflate (reduced compliance)

High peak inspiratory pressures (PIP) cause alveolar damage, 'barotrauma' and pneumothorax in normal lung tissue
Use low PIP (<30 cmH_2O)

(d) V/Q matching

1. PEEP: recruits collapsed alveoli

2. Nitric oxide

NO

NO

Consolidated alveoli

NO increases blood flow past ventilated alveoli

Reduces shunt

3. Prone position

Back

Consolidated lung

Normal lung

Front

Blood flow greatest in dependent lung

↓

V/Q matching improved

(c) Common causes of ARDS

Direct pulmonary	Indirect
Infective (pneumonia, tuberculosis)	Sepsis
Pulmonary trauma	Non-thoracic trauma
Near-drowning	Burns
Toxic gas inhalation	Haemorrhage, multiple transfusion
Smoke	Post arrest
NO_2, NH_3, Cl_2	Bowel infarction
Phosgene	Anaphylactic
Oxygen toxicity ($F_iO_2 >0.8$)	Pancreatitis
Inhalation of gastric contents (pH <2)	Uraemia, toxins, eclampsia
	Drugs (salicylates, barbiturates)

Acute respiratory distress syndrome (ARDS) is most simply defined as 'leaky lung syndrome' or 'low-pressure (i.e. non-cardiogenic) pulmonary oedema'. It describes an acute, diffuse inflammatory lung injury, often in previously healthy lungs (Fig. 41a) in response to a variety of direct (i.e. inhaled) or indirect (i.e. bloodborne) insults.

The **internationally agreed criteria** for diagnosis of ARDS are:
1 Severe hypoxaemia, P_aO_2/F_iO_2 <200, (±positive end-expiratory pressure (PEEP)), e.g. P_aO_2 (55 mmHg)/F_iO_2 (80% inspired O_2) = 55/0.8 = 75
2 Bilateral diffuse pulmonary infiltrates on chest X-ray
3 Normal or only slightly elevated left atrial pressure (pulmonary artery occlusion pressure <18 mmHg).

Acute lung injury (ALI) is the precursor to ARDS. Apart from a lesser degree of hypoxaemia (P_aO_2/F_iO_2 <300), the criteria for diagnosis are the same.

Epidemiology and prognosis

The **incidence** of ARDS is approximately 2–8 cases per 100 000 population per year, but its precursor ALI is much more common. ARDS mortality is generally **high (>40%)** but is determined by the precipitating condition (~35% for trauma, ~50% for sepsis and ~80% for aspiration pneumonia). Age (>60 years) and sepsis are also associated with increased mortality. Early diagnosis and treatment may improve outcome. The cause of death is **multiorgan failure (MOF)**, usually due to a combination of tissue hypoxia and overwhelming secondary infection. Less than 20% of patients die from hypoxaemia alone.

Pathogenesis (Fig. 41a and b) and causes (Fig. 41c)

During the **acute inflammatory phase** of ARDS, cytokine-activated neutrophils and monocytes adhere to pulmonary endothelium or alveolar epithelium, releasing inflammatory mediators and proteolytic enzymes (Chapter 18). These damage the integrity of the alveolar–capillary membrane, increase permeability and cause alveolar oedema. Reduced surfactant production causes alveolar collapse and hyaline membrane formation. The loss of functioning alveoli and ventilation/perfusion mismatch leads to progressive hypoxaemia and respiratory failure. The subsequent late **healing fibroproliferative phase** results in progressive pulmonary fibrosis and reduced compliance (stiff lungs). Associated pulmonary hypertension is partially due to activation of the coagulation cascade, with pulmonary capillary microthrombosis and regional hypoxic vasoconstriction.

Clinical features

The **acute inflammatory phase** lasts 3–10 days and results in hypoxaemia and MOF. It presents with progressive breathlessness, tachypnoea, central cyanosis, hypoxic confusion and lung crepitations. These symptoms and signs are in no way diagnostic and are shared with many other pulmonary conditions. During the later **healing, fibroproliferative phase**, pulmonary fibrosis (lung scarring) and pneumothoraxes (Chapter 35) are common. Secondary chest and systemic infections complicate both phases.

Investigations

Monitoring: Routine measurements include temperature, respiratory rate, O_2 saturation and urine output. In addition, the arterial and central venous pressures, the cardiac output and occasionally the left atrial pressure (using a pulmonary artery catheter) are measured **to assess fluid balance and ensure adequate tissue oxygen delivery**. Serial blood gas measurements are used to monitor gas exchange. Early detection of secondary pulmonary infection requires microbiological examination of sputum or bronchoalveolar lavage.

Radiological: Serial chest X-rays (CXRs) identify progression of **diffuse bilateral pulmonary infiltrates**. Similarly, early computed tomography (CT) scanning can identify **diffuse patchy infiltrates** with **dependent consolidation**; later scans reveal **pneumothoraxes, pneumatoceles** and **fibrosis**.

Management

The key to successful management of ARDS is to **establish and treat the underlying cause**. In the early stages, oxygen therapy and physiotherapy may suffice. With progressive respiratory failure, non-invasive ventilation – with continuous positive airway pressure (CPAP) or non-invasive positive pressure ventilation (NIPPV) – or full mechanical ventilation and high-inspired oxygen concentrations may be required to maintain adequate ventilation and oxygenation. The high airways pressures needed to achieve normal tidal volumes during mechanical ventilation often result in lung damage (barotrauma), including pneumothorax and lung cysts. This ventilator-induced lung injury and oxygen toxicity (F_iO_2 >0.8) must be prevented, as these contribute to mortality and multiorgan failure (Fig. 41b).

The basic principles of mechanical ventilation are to **limit pressure-induced damage, optimize oxygenation** and **avoid circulatory compromise** (reduced cardiac output and blood pressure due to high intrathoracic pressures; see also Chapter 42). A 'protective lung ventilation strategy' of low tidal volumes (6 mL/kg) and low peak inspiratory pressures (<30 cmH$_2$O) reduces lung damage, complications and mortality. **Alveolar recruitment** (of collapsed alveoli) is achieved with high positive end-expiratory pressures (PEEP >10 cmH$_2$O) or long inspiratory–expiratory times. The CO_2 retention ('permissive hypercapnia') resulting from this strategy of low tidal volume ventilation can be tolerated for long periods.

Excessive fluid loading must be avoided, as this increases the alveolar flooding characteristic of ARDS. The aim must be to maintain adequate perfusion of other organs while using the lowest possible left atrial pressures. In the acute situation, diuretics may be essential to correct hypoxaemia by reducing extravascular lung water. Thereafter, combinations of systemic vasodilators (after load reduction of the left heart), inotropes and vasoconstrictor agents may be used to achieve adequate cardiac output and perfusion pressures at low left atrial filling pressures.

Essential general measures include good nursing care, physiotherapy, nutrition and infection control. Reducing fever (shivering) and controlling anxiety with sedation decrease metabolic demand. **No drug therapy has been consistently beneficial** in early ARDS, including steroids, anti-inflammatory agents, anticytokines or surfactant therapy. However, 7–10 days after onset, steroid therapy may prevent the development of subsequent pulmonary fibrosis. **Inhaled nitric oxide** and nursing the patient in the **prone position** improve gas exchange by increasing perfusion to ventilated areas of lung, but no survival benefit has been demonstrated (Fig. 41d). **Extracorporeal membrane oxygenation (ECMO)** techniques to oxygenate blood or remove CO_2 are effective in children, but the benefit in adults has not been established.

(a) Indications for mechanical ventilation or support in adults

Surgery General anaesthesia with neuromuscular blockade Postoperative management following major surgery	**Cervical cord damage above C4** Neck fractures
Respiratory centre depression Usually when P_aCO_2 >7–8 kPa (50–60 mmHg) Head injury Drug overdose, e.g. opiates, barbiturates Raised intracranial pressure: cerebral haemorrhage/ tumours/meningitis/encephalitis Status epilepticus	**Neuromuscular disorders** when VC <20–30 mL/kg Guillain–Barré Myasthenia gravis Poliomyelitis Polyneuritis
	Chest wall disorders Kyphoscoliosis Trauma: especially flail segment (multiple rib fractures → section of chest wall unattached)
Lung disease Pneumonia Acute respiratory distress syndrome (ARDS) Severe asthma attack Acute exacerbation of chronic obstructive pulmonary disease (COPD), cystic fibrosis Trauma–lung contusion Pulmonary oedema	**Other** Cardiac arrest Severe circulatory shock Resistant hypoxia in type 1 respiratory failure (reduces oxygen consumption)

(c) Airway pressure profiles in different types of ventilation

(b) Nasal mask and NIPPV

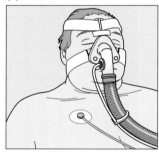

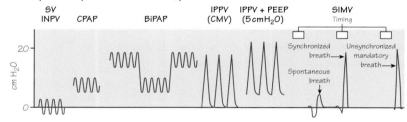

SV = spontaneous ventilation, **INPV** = intermittent negative pressure ventilation, **CPAP** = continuous positive airway pressure, **BiPAP** = biphasic continuous airway pressure (trace shown is fixed time period BiPAP), **IPPV** = intermittent positive pressure ventilation (= CMV), **CMV** = controlled mechanical ventilation, **PEEP** = positive end-expiratory pressure, **SIMV** = synchronized intermittent mandatory ventilation. If a spontaneous breath occurs in the timing window it triggers a synchronized ventilator breath and if not a mandatory breath is given soon after the timing window.

(d) Complications of mechanical ventilation

Risks during endotracheal intubation or tracheostomy Myocardial depression from anaesthetic Aspiration of gastric contents Fall in P_aO_2 during apnoea Reflex bronchoconstriction and laryngospasm	*Risks associated with sedation and paralysis* Cardiac depression Depression of respiratory drive (delays weaning) Increases danger of disconnection/ventilator failure
Risks of endotracheal intubation and tracheostomy Intubation of the oesophagus Intubation of a bronchus Blockage/accidental extubation Laryngeal/tracheal damage or stenosis Infection	*Risks associated with mechanical ventilation* High airway pressure → barotrauma Alveolar overdistension → volutrauma: • Pneumothorax, pneumomediastinum • Subcutaneous emphysema (= air in skin) • Structural damage to lung, airways and capillaries • Bronchopulmonary dysplasia (see Chapter 17)
Risks associated with high inspired oxygen (see Chapter 43)	

Mechanical ventilation is usually used to prevent or treat type 2 respiratory (ventilatory) failure. The main indications in adults are listed in Fig. 42a.

Types of mechanical ventilation
(Fig. 42c)

Inspiratory muscle paralysis by poliomyelitis was a common reason for mechanical ventilation in the first half of the twentieth century. It was usually performed by **intermittent negative pressure ventilation (INPV)**, which is still occasionally used today. Patients are placed inside a **tank ventilator** sealed at the neck, and tank pressure is intermittently lowered, expanding the chest and lowering intrapleural pressure as in spontaneous breathing. Disadvantages of this **iron lung** include claustrophobia, discomfort, difficult nursing care and the bulk and expense of the equipment. **Jacket** and **cuirass ventilators** produce a negative pressure just around the chest, but difficulty in achieving a satisfactory seal limits their use to patients only needing ventilatory augmentation.

From the 1950s, **intermittent positive pressure ventilation (IPPV; controlled mechanical ventilation, CMV)** quickly replaced INPV for most purposes. Air is driven into the lungs by raising airway pressure, usually via an endotracheal or tracheostomy tube. Expiration is achieved by allowing pressure to fall to zero. This simple form of IPPV is used during routine surgery. Typical initial adult settings for IPPV are:

Tidal volume, $V_T = 8–12$ mL/kg

Respiratory frequency, $f = 8–14$ breaths/min

Minute ventilation, $V(= V_T \times f) \approx 6000$ mL/min

Inspiratory time/expiratory time $= 1 : 2–1 : 3$

Minute ventilation is adjusted to maintain P_aCO_2 at about 5 kPa (37 mmHg). A slightly lower P_aCO_2 may be used initially in the presence of raised intracranial pressure. Accepting a higher P_aCO_2 (**permissive hypercapnia**) may prevent the need for excessively high airway pressures. P_aO_2 is maintained above 10 kPa (75 mmHg) by adjusting inspired FO_2. The lowest concentration needed is used, usually in the range 30–60%. It may be preferable to accept a slightly lower PO_2 than to use more than 60% for long periods.

Microprocessor control of ventilators has permitted development of numerous variations of IPPV. For example, in non-paralysed patients, the positive pressure may be synchronized with spontaneous breaths and a mandatory breath given if no spontaneous breaths occur in a preset time (**synchronized intermittent mandatory ventilation, SIMV**). In another form, the ventilator operates only where spontaneous ventilation falls below a preset minimum (**mandatory minute ventilation, MMV**).

If, instead of allowing airway pressure to fall to zero, a small positive pressure is maintained throughout expiration (**positive end-expiratory pressure, PEEP**), there is a reduction in V_A/Q mismatching and an improvement in P_aO_2 in some conditions, such as acute respiratory distress syndrome (ARDS). This occurs because PEEP increases functional residual capacity (FRC) and reduces the closure of airways and alveoli towards the end of expiration. Unfortunately, intrathoracic pressure is raised, impairing venous return, and occasionally the fall in cardiac output can reduce tissue oxygen delivery despite the increased P_aO_2.

The increased mean airway pressure caused by PEEP also increases the risk of barotrauma. A good compromise is to use the minimum PEEP required to keep PO_2 at an acceptable level (>8 kPa, 60 mmHg) when breathing 50–60% oxygen.

Non-invasive respiratory support

Non-invasive ventilation avoids the use of tracheal intubation or tracheostomy. An example is INPV (above), but this is no longer widely used. In contrast, non-invasive positive pressure techniques using either a nasal mask (Fig. 42b) or sometimes a full face mask are increasingly being used.

In **continuous positive airway pressure (CPAP)**, a standing pressure of 5–10 cmH$_2$O is applied to a nasal or face mask in a spontaneously breathing patient (Fig. 42c). This has several potential beneficial effects. First, it helps prevent upper airway collapse in **obstructive sleep apnoea**. In interstitial diseases such as **ARDS**, it recruits alveoli, reducing V_A/Q mismatching. FRC is increased, and this may increase lung compliance by moving the patient onto the steep part of the pressure–volume curve (Chapter 6). CO_2 retention may be a problem during CPAP, which may be improved by using biphasic or bilevel positive pressure ventilation (BiPAP). BiPAP alternates between high and low pressure either for fixed time periods (Fig. 42c) or between inspiration and expiration, making expiration easier and improving the emptying of the lungs.

CPAP may improve oxygenation and may aid the patient's own respiratory efforts, but it cannot produce ventilation by itself. In contrast, **non-invasive intermittent positive pressure ventilation (NIPPV)** is IPPV delivered by face or, more usually, nasal mask. For it to be used successfully, the patient must be cooperative and introduced to the technique gradually, to allow synchronization of his or her breathing with the ventilator. Its use includes nocturnal ventilation of patients with chronic respiratory failure due to neuromuscular disease or thoracic deformity. It is well established for the treatment of respiratory failure caused by acute exacerbations of chronic obstructive pulmonary disease (COPD), avoiding the need for intubation and improving survival. It is increasingly being used for a range of other conditions as an alternative to standard IPPV.

In summary, the main beneficial effect of **CPAP** is recruitment of alveoli. The reduction in collapse sometimes also gives rise to a reduction in the work of breathing. In contrast, **NIPPV** is used to reduce or take over the work of breathing rather than to recruit alveoli. This may be of benefit in the tired (e.g. COPD) patient.

Weaning the patient off the ventilator following surgery is usually achieved by reversing neuromuscular blockade and lightening the anaesthetic level. In ICU patients, weaning may be more difficult. Several techniques are used, including removing mechanical ventilation for progressively longer periods, or by using a spontaneously breathing mode (e.g. SIMV), and pressure support in which support is progressively reduced. CPAP applied via the endotracheal tube may also help the weaning process.

Problems are hard to predict accurately, but are most likely following prolonged ventilation, in debilitated patients, or in those with neuromuscular or chronic respiratory disease. A pattern of rapid shallow breathing 5 minutes after disconnection from the ventilator is one of the more useful predictors of failure.

Complications of mechanical ventilation are numerous, and are listed in Fig. 42d.

43 Oxygenation and oxygen therapy

(a) Indications for acute oxygen therapy

1. Cardiac and respiratory arrest
2. Hypoxaemia (P_aO_2 <8kPa, S_aO_2 <90%)
3. Hypotension (systolic BP <100 mmHg)
4. Low cardiac output
5. Metabolic acidosis (bicarbonate <18 mmol/L)
6. Respiratory distress (respiratory rate >24/min)

(c) Risks associated with high-dose oxygen therapy

1. **Carbon dioxide retention:**
   ~10% of breathless patients, mainly COPD, have type 2 respiratory failure (RF). ~40–50% of COPD patients are at risk of type 2 RF
2. **Rebound hypoxaemia:**
   occurs if oxygen is suddenly withdrawn in type 2 RF
3. **Absorption collapse**
   O_2 in poorly ventilated alveoli is rapidly absorbed whereas N_2 absorption is slow, so high FO_2 can cause collapse
4. **Pulmonary oxygen toxicity**
   F_iO_2>60% may damage alveolar membranes causing ARDS if inhaled for >24–48 hrs (Chapter 41). Hyperoxia can cause coronary and cerebral vasospasm
5. **Fire**
   Deaths and burns occur in smokers during O_2 therapy
6. **Paul–Bert effect**
   Hyperbaric O_2 can cause cerebral vasoconstriction and epileptic fits

(d) Oxygen delivery devices

1. Variable performance devices

Air is entrained during breathing whilst oxygen is delivered from a reservoir (i.e. mask, reservoir bag, nasopharynx)

The F_iO_2 delivered to the lungs depends on the oxygen flow rate, the patient's inspiratory flow, respiratory rate and the amount of air entrained

e.g. Figure (i) 'Low-flow face masks', O_2 flows at ~2–10 L/min into the mask and is supplemented by air drawn into the mask. The F_iO_2 achieved depends on ventilation

Ventilation = 5 L/min

O_2 flow = 2 L/min; air (21% O_2) flow = 3 L/min
F_iO_2 = (2+0.21 x 3)/5 x 100 = **53%**

Ventilation = 25 L/min

O_2 flow = 2 L/min; air (21% O_2) flow = 23 L/min
F_iO_2 = (2+0.21 x 23)/25 x 100 = **27%**

These devices cannot be used if accurate control of F_iO_2 is desirable, e.g. COPD with hypercapnia

Examples of variable performance devices are 'low-flow' facemasks (see i), nasal cannulae (see ii) and non-rebreathing face masks with reservoir bags (see iii)

2. Fixed performance devices

Are independent of the patient's pattern of breathing and inspiratory volume

Figure (iv) illustrates that a fixed O_2 flow through a Venturi valve entrains the correct proportion of air to achieve the required O_2 concentration

This system delivers more gas than is inspired (i.e. >30 L/min). Consequently, F_iO_2 is less affected by the breathing pattern. The resulting masks are high flow, low concentration and fixed performance

Used in patients with COPD and respiratory failure to avoid CO_2 retention

(i) 'Low-flow' facemask

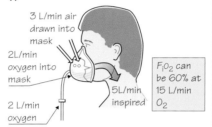

3 L/min air drawn into mask
2L/min oxygen into mask
2 L/min oxygen
5L/min inspired

F_iO_2 can be 60% at 15 L/min O_2

O_2 flows at ~2–15 L/min into the mask and is supplemented by air drawn into the mask. Flow rate must be > 5 L/min to prevent CO_2 rebreathing

(ii) Nasal cannulae

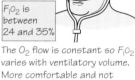

O_2 flow rates up to 4 L/min. Higher rates dry mucosa

F_iO_2 is between 24 and 35%

The O_2 flow is constant so F_iO_2 varies with ventilatory volume. More comfortable and not removed during eating or coughing.
O_2 inhaled even when mouth breathing

(iii) Non-rebreathing and anaesthetic masks

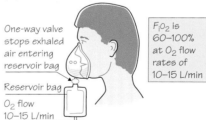

One-way valve stops exhaled air entering reservoir bag
Reservoir bag
O_2 flow 10–15 L/min

F_iO_2 is 60–100% at O_2 flow rates of 10–15 L/min

High (10–15 L/min) flow rates of O_2 provide high F_iO_2 > 60% and up to 100%

Non-rebreathing masks have a reservoir bag which should be filled before use. They increase F_iO_2 by preventing O_2 loss during expiration

(iv) 'High-flow' (Venturi), low concentration face mask

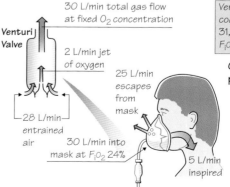

30 L/min total gas flow at fixed O_2 concentration
Venturi Valve
2 L/min jet of oxygen
25 L/min escapes from mask
28 L/min entrained air
30 L/min into mask at F_iO_2 24%
5 L/min inspired

Venturi valves are colour coded and deliver 24, 28, 31, 35, 40 or 60% F_iO_2 for a fixed flow rate

Continuous positive airways pressure (CPAP) masks
Use a tight fitting mask and a flow generator to deliver a fixed F_iO_2 with a positive pressure (5–10 cm/H_2O) throughout the respiratory cycle

Sufficient O_2 must be delivered to the tissues to support metabolism, and the tissues must be able to utilize it. **Tissue hypoxia** can be caused by **low arterial P_{O_2}** and therefore **blood O_2 content** (hypoxaemia); inadequate **tissue blood flow** (ischaemia, cardiac failure, emboli); low **haemoglobin concentration** (anaemia); abnormal **oxygen dissociation curve** (haemoglobinopathies, CO poisoning); and **poisoning of intracellular oxygen usage** (e.g. cyanide and sepsis). Tissue hypoxia occurs within 4 minutes of failure of any of these systems because tissue and lung O_2 reserves are small. Clinical features are often non-specific, including altered mental state, dyspnoea, hyperventilation, arrhythmias and hypotension (see Chapter 23). Anaemia and abnormal dissociation curves are discussed in Chapter 8.

Measuring tissue hypoxia

Arterial oxygen saturation (S_aO_2) is measured with a **pulse oximeter**, and partial pressure of oxygen (P_aO_2) by **blood gas analysis**. SaO_2 should be measured regularly in all breathless patients. However, both P_aO_2 and S_aO_2 can be normal when tissue hypoxia is caused by low cardiac output states, anaemia and failure of tissue O_2 use. In these circumstances, **mixed venous oxygen partial pressure** ($P_v−O_2$), which is measured in blood taken from a pulmonary artery catheter, approximates to mean tissue P_{O_2}. However, severe hypoxia in a single organ (e.g. due to an arterial embolus) may be associated with a normal P_aO_2, S_aO_2 and P_vO_2.

Oxygen therapy

Given correctly O_2 is a lifesaving drug, but it is often used without appropriate evaluation of potential benefits and side effects. Figure 43a lists indications for initiating O_2 therapy, whereas Figure 43b lists potential risks. Immediate assessment of airways, breathing and circulation is essential to confirm airway patency and good circulation. Figure 43c illustrates important features of O_2 delivery systems. The aims of O_2 therapy depend on the risk of developing **type 2 (hypercapnic, CO_2 retaining) respiratory failure** (Chapter 23):

- **In normal patients** (low risk of type 2 respiratory failure) aim for an SaO_2 of 94–98% (92–98% if >70 years), i.e. the plateau of the O_2–haemoglobin dissociation curve; increasing PaO_2 further has no impact on O_2 delivery as little O_2 is dissolved in plasma (Chapter 8).
- **In patients at risk of type 2 respiratory failure** (e.g. COPD) target SaO_2 should be 88–92% pending arterial blood gas (ABG) analysis. A higher SaO_2 has few advantages but results in hypoventilation, hypercapnia and respiratory acidosis in patients dependent on hypoxic respiratory drive (Chapter 11).

Initial O_2 dose and delivery method depends on cause of hypoxia:

- **High-dose supplemental oxygen** (>60%) is delivered through a non-rebreathing, reservoir mask at 10–15 L/min (Fig. 43c(iii)). Indicating conditions include cardiac or respiratory arrest, shock, major trauma, sepsis, CO poisoning and critical illness. Once the patient is stable, the O_2 dose is reduced to maintain an SaO_2 of 92–98%. Seriously ill patients at risk of hypercapnic respiratory failure (HCRF) are initially treated with high-dose O_2 pending ABG analysis.

- **Moderate-dose supplemental oxygen** (40–60%) is given in serious illnesses (e.g. pneumonia) through nasal cannulae (2–6 L/min) or simple face masks (5–10 L/min), aiming for an SaO_2 of 92–98% (Fig. 43c(i,ii)). A reservoir mask is substituted if this is not achieved.
- **Low-dose (controlled) supplemental oxygen** (24–28%) is delivered through a fixed performance Venturi mask (Fig. 43c(iv)). It is indicated in patients at risk of **CO_2 retaining, type 2 respiratory failure**, including COPD, neuromuscular disease, chest wall disorders and cystic fibrosis. Target SaO_2 is 88–92% whilst awaiting ABG results. If P_aCO_2 is normal, the SaO_2 is adjusted to 92–98% (except in patients with previous type 2 respiratory failure) and ABG rechecked at 1 hour. A raised P_aCO_2 and bicarbonate with normal pH suggest longstanding hypercapnia and type 2 respiratory failure (Chapter 10); the target SaO_2 should therefore be 88–92% with repeat ABG at 1 hour. If the patient is hypercapnic (P_aCO_2 >6 kPa) and acidotic (pH <7.35), non-invasive ventilation (NIV, Chapter 42) should be considered. Venturi masks are replaced with nasal cannulae (1–2 L/min) when the patient is stable. An O_2 alert card and Venturi mask are issued to patients with previous type 2 respiratory failure to warn future emergency staff of the potential risk.

Oxygen therapy is of little benefit in 'normoxic' patients because the haemoglobin is fully saturated. Restoration of tissue blood flow is often more important in these cases. In myocardial infarction, drug overdoses, metabolic disorders, hyperventilation or during labour in non-hypoxic pregnant women, O_2 therapy is of little value. It may actually be harmful in normoxic patients with strokes, paraquat poisoning or acid inhalation, and to the fetus in normoxic obstetric emergencies. However, in **CO poisoning** high-dose O_2 is essential, despite a normal PaO_2, to reduce the half-life of carboxyhaemoglobin (Chapter 8).

Stop oxygen therapy when the patient is clinically stable on low-dose O_2 (e.g. 1–2 L/min) and SaO_2 is within the desired range on two consecutive occasions. Monitor SaO_2 for 5 minutes after stopping O_2 and recheck at 1 hour.

Other techniques to improve oxygenation

1 **Anaemia:** Failure of tissue O_2 delivery is best corrected by blood transfusion.

2 **Block of airways by mucus and retention of secretions** (e.g. cystic fibrosis, Chapter 34) requires physiotherapy, mucolytic agents and occasionally bronchoscopy to remove blockages and improve alveolar ventilation.

3 **Fluid restriction** reduces alveolar oedema when alveolar permeability is increased (e.g. ARDS, Chapter 41).

4 **Alveolar recruitment** improves oxygenation by reducing V_A/Q mismatch and shunt (Chapters 13 and 14). Simple postural changes may improve oxygenation. Sitting upright optimizes V_A/Q matching in the alert patient. Regular turning and prone positioning improve secretion drainage and oxygenation in supine patients. Techniques that increase mean alveolar pressures (e.g. PEEP, CPAP and increased inspiratory/expiratory ratio) also improve alveolar recruitment and oxygenation (Chapters 42).

5 **Ventilatory support** (e.g. NIV) improves oxygenation by correcting hypoventilation and associated hypercapnia (Chapters 9 and 42).

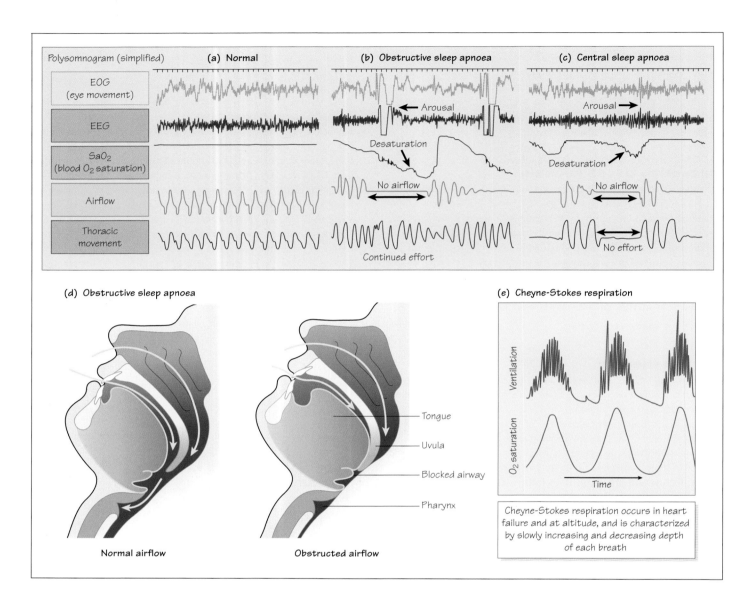

Polysomnogram (simplified)

(a) Normal   **(b) Obstructive sleep apnoea**   **(c) Central sleep apnoea**

EOG (eye movement)

EEG

SaO₂ (blood O₂ saturation)

Airflow

Thoracic movement

Arousal — Arousal

Desaturation   Desaturation

No airflow   No airflow

Continued effort   No effort

(d) Obstructive sleep apnoea

Tongue
Uvula
Blocked airway
Pharynx

Normal airflow   Obstructed airflow

(e) Cheyne-Stokes respiration

Ventilation

O₂ saturation

Time

Cheyne-Stokes respiration occurs in heart failure and at altitude, and is characterized by slowly increasing and decreasing depth of each breath

Sleep apnoea (or sleep-disordered breathing) is common, with a vast potential for improvement in quality of life. It is caused by obstruction of the upper airways (**obstructive sleep apnoea**), and more rarely **central sleep apnoea (CSA)**, where the central control of ventilation is disturbed. It can lead to significant sleep deprivation and fragmentation and thus daytime hypersomnolence (sleepiness), with consequent decreased quality of life, mental and physical performance, and increased risk of accidents and cardiovascular disease, such as hypertension. Sleep-disordered breathing is diagnosed using **polysomnography** (Fig. 44a), which records the electroencephalography (EEG) for sleep patterns, movements of abdomen and thorax to assess breathing, oronasal flow and oximetry for O_2 saturation. Normal sleep (Fig. 44a) consists of rapid eye movement (**REM**, $\sim$25%) and non-rapid eye movement (**NREM**) sleep. REM sleep is characterized by an awake-pattern EEG, voluntary muscle atonia and dreaming. Ventilatory drive is normally diminished in REM sleep, causing a slight fall in P_aO_2 and a rise in P_aCO_2. Sleep apnoea is associated with multiple periods of hypoxaemia and partial awakenings (Fig. 44b and c).

Obstructive sleep apnoea

Obstructive sleep apnoea (OSA) is characterized by absence of airflow with continued respiratory effort (Fig. 44b). About 90% of patients with sleep apnoea have OSA. OSA is far more common in males than females, and is associated with alcohol consumption, increasing age, obesity, increased neck circumference, hypertension and hypothyroidism. Obstruction typically occurs in the upper airway and pharynx, and is related to the normal decrease in upper airway muscle tone that occurs in REM sleep coupled with narrowing of the pharyngeal airways due to obesity or enlarged tonsils. Neuromuscular disease (e.g. stroke) and muscle relaxants (e.g. alcohol and sedatives) may further reduce upper airway muscle tone. These factors, in conjunction with individual anatomy and posture, result in airway obstruction during inspiration, when airway pressure is reduced (Fig. 44d).

Apnoea resolves with arousal and restoration of muscle tone. Although hundreds or thousands of episodes of apnoea and arousal may occur each night in severe cases, patients are often unaware of them; sleep partners commonly report **loud snoring**, snorting or apnoea. Patients commonly report unrefreshing sleep and nocturia, develop **daytime hypersomnolence** and **gain weight**, and may show pedal oedema, nasal congestion, enlarged tongue, shallow palate, enlarged uvula or retrognathia. Most patients have normal arterial blood gases and haemoglobin. In chronic obstructive pulmonary disease (COPD), **nocturnal hypoxia** can be severe even with mild OSA, as gas exchange is already compromised.

Polysomnography reveals repeated episodes of OSA or hypopnoea (reduced airflow with oxygen desaturation or arousal), which terminate with arousal (Fig. 44b). These episodes are quantified by the **apnoea plus hypopnoea index** (**AHI**, episodes/hour). Normal sleep has an AHI of less than 10. Severe OSA usually has an AHI of more than 40. A minority of patients with very severe OSA may develop **obesity hy-**poventilation syndrome (Pickwick syndrome). Obstructive episodes can cause **pulmonary hypertension** (Chapter 27) from hypoxic pulmonary vasoconstriction. Systemic blood pressure increases during apnoea, possibly due to sympathetic stimulation, and left ventricle (LV) afterload increases during obstructive apnoeas due to the marked fall in pleural pressure. There is a strong association between OSA and systemic hypertension, although the cause is unknown.

Therapy requires relief of obstruction. Moderate weight loss ($\geq$10%) often results in substantial improvements, as does limiting evening consumption of alcohol. When OSA is significant, **nasal continuous positive airway pressure** (**CPAP**, Chapter 42) is the most commonly prescribed therapy, but 50% of patients do not comply in the long term. Some patients respond to oral appliances or removal of tonsils, though uvulopalatopharyngoplasty (surgery) is rarely beneficial. O_2 alone may decrease or eliminate hypoxia, but not the obstruction or arousals.

Central sleep apnoea

CSA is characterized by cessation of airflow during sleep without evidence of respiratory effort, and is due to a **loss or inhibition of central respiratory drive** (Fig. 44c). Patients with CSA may be subdivided into those with daytime hypercapnia or normocapnia. CSA with daytime hypercapnia is usually due to central alveolar hypoventilation, neuromuscular disease or restrictive chest wall disease (e.g. kyphoscoliosis). Central alveolar hypoventilation may be congenital or due to brainstem disease and strokes (see also Ondine's curse; Chapter 12). Neuromuscular causes include muscular dystrophy, phrenic nerve dysfunction, myositis (muscle inflammation) and myasthenia gravis. Inspiratory muscle impairment in restrictive or obstructive (e.g. COPD) respiratory disease can lead to increased use of accessory muscles during ventilation, but voluntary muscle atonia during REM sleep can therefore lead to profound hypoxaemia.

Cheyne-Stokes respiration is an abnormal pattern of breathing characterized by gradual waxing and waning of the depth of breathing, leading to periods of hypoventilation and desaturation (Fig. 44d). It is commonly experienced in patients with heart failure and at altitude. The underlying causes are not fully understood, but may include dysregulation of feedback from the chemoreceptors (Chapter 11). Under these conditions hypoxaemia can lead to hyperventilation and thus hypocapnia and alkalosis. On sleeping, ventilatory drive may be depressed, leading to hypercapnia or apnoea and hypoxaemia, which causes arousal and hyperventilation again, and the sequence repeats throughout the sleeping period.

Therapy for CSA depends on symptoms. Patients with a CNS cause for hypoventilation ('won't breathe') may benefit from a respiratory stimulant. Patients with weakness or chest wall disease ('can't breathe') benefit from assisted mechanical ventilation, specifically non-invasive intermittent positive pressure ventilation (**NIPPV**, Chapter 42). Cheyne-Stokes respiration can be improved by treatment of the underlying condition (heart failure) or raising the inspired O_2.

Case studies: questions

Case 1

At the start of your shift on an orthopaedic ward, you are asked to review two patients.

Elizabeth is a 70-year-old who was making a good recovery from her hip replacement 3 days ago. This morning while eating breakfast, she developed sudden breathlessness. She denies any pain.

Alice is a 35-year-old woman who had an internal fixation of a femoral shaft fracture following a road traffic accident 4 days earlier. This morning she complains of pleuritic pain but no breathlessness.

Initial clinical findings for Elizabeth are blood pressure (BP) of 110/80 mmHg, heart rate (HR) 95 beats/min, respiratory rate 24 breaths/min and oxygen saturation 86%. Initial clinical findings for Alice are BP 126/80 mmHg, HR 80 beats/min, respiratory rate 18 breaths/min and oxygen saturation 97%.

In both patients, examination is otherwise unremarkable and the initial chest X-ray and electrocardiogram (ECG) are normal, although a repeat X-ray the following day shows that Alice has developed a small right-sided pleural effusion.

Questions

1 *You are worried whether either or both could have a pulmonary embolus (PE). From the history and findings so far, is this likely in either or both of these patients? If these patients had not had surgery recently but had presented with the same symptoms and signs in Accident and Emergency, would your answer be different?*

2 *Which of these oxygen saturations is 'typical' of a pulmonary embolus?*

3 *Pulmonary emboli produce an area of lung that is ventilated but not perfused; that is, they produce alveolar dead space and therefore increase physiological dead space. Does increased physiological dead space inevitably lead to a reduced arterial P_{O_2}?*

4 *What other aspects of the history might be relevant?*

5 *D-dimer tests are a useful addition to the diagnostic armoury but false-positives are common. False-negatives also occur. Which sort of PE is most likely to be associated with a false-negative PE? How long do D-dimers remain elevated?*

6 *What is the role of chest X-ray (CXR) and electrocardiogram (ECG)? How will they be affected in the presence of a pulmonary embolus?*

7 *What other investigations are appropriate?*

8 *What are the treatment options for Elizabeth and Alice?*

Case 2

Tom, who is 15 years old, attends his general practitioner's (GP) asthma clinic. He has had asthma since early childhood. On two occasions, when he was 8 and 10 years old, he had attacks severe enough to require hospital admission. At present, his asthma is well controlled on regular inhaled beclometasone dipropionate, 200 µg twice daily, and inhaled salmeterol, 50 µg twice daily. Today, his peak flow is 510 L/min (predicted value for his age and height 530 L/min). On auscultation, there is vesicular breathing and no other sounds.

Questions

1 *Is this peak flow normal? Apart from the nomogram values, can you think of any other peak flow reading with which it would be useful to compare today's clinic reading?*

2 *If you measured the following:*
- *FEV_1/FVC*
- *Airway resistance*
- *Functional residual capacity (FRC)*
- *Lung compliance*
- *Arterial P_{O_2} and arterial P_{CO_2}*

– how would they compare with the normal for a boy of his age and size?

On a school trip to a countryside park, Tom becomes breathless running across a field. His teacher is alarmed by his noisy breathing and asks you, a passing medical student, to assess whether they need to get him to hospital.

3 *What simple observations can you make that will help you decide how severe this attack is? In his backpack he has a salbutamol inhaler, a salmeterol inhaler, a sodium cromoglycate inhaler and a beclometasone inhaler. Which should he use?*

4 *If you had been able to measure the following during his episode of breathlessness:*
- *FEV_1/FVC*
- *Peak flow rate*
- *Airway resistance*
- *Functional residual capacity*
- *Lung compliance*
- *Arterial P_{O_2} and arterial P_{CO_2}*

– how do you think they would compare with the normal for a boy of his age and size?

5 *If you had had your stethoscope with you, what would you have heard on examining his chest?*

At 18 years of age, Tom goes to college in London. He stops taking regular medication, as he feels he has 'grown out' of his asthma. He keeps a salbutamol inhaler in his room 'just in case'. During the first term he is well, apart from a couple of wheezy episodes while playing football. In the second term, he develops a heavy cold, and over 24 hours he becomes progressively more breathless despite frequent puffs of salbutamol. His friends call out his GP, who finds the following: Tom is fully alert, but talking in broken sentences because he is very breathless. He is not cyanosed. He is using his accessory muscles of respiration. On auscultation, there are widespread expiratory rhonchi (wheezes). BP is 115/80 mmHg, HR 110 beats/min, respiratory rate 30 breaths/min, peak flow 200 L/min.

6 *Which observations suggest that this is a fairly severe attack?*

7 *If the GP had measured airway resistance, FRC, lung compliance, arterial P_{O_2} and P_{CO_2}, how would they compare to the predicted values?*

His GP decides that this attack warrants hospital admission, and he calls an ambulance. Unfortunately, owing to heavy traffic it is 40 minutes before he arrives at the local Accident and Emergency department. By this time, Tom is confused, too breathless to talk and unable to produce a peak flow reading. The Accident and Emergency *officer notices he is now cyanosed, although the widespread rhonchi noted in the GP's letter have now disappeared. Arterial blood gases show arterial $P_{O_2} = 7$ kPa and arterial $P_{CO_2} = 5.5$ kPa while breathing 60% oxygen.*

8 Discuss the features that suggest this asthma attack is life-threatening. Do the reduced rhonchi on auscultation contradict the other findings?

9 What is the cause of the low arterial P_{O_2}? Was the inhaled oxygen helpful, and if so was the correct concentration used? Is this P_{CO_2} normal, and how does it affect your assessment of the severity of this attack?

Case 3

A 38-year-old man is seen for evaluation of severe exertional dyspnoea. Two years ago, he had been able to play squash regularly, but he stopped 6 months ago because of dyspnoea and fatigue during exercise. He now reports dyspnoea after climbing one flight of stairs. He has no cough, sputum or wheeze. He smoked one pack of cigarettes a day for 10 years and quit 7 years ago. He has no allergies or pets, and has not travelled outside Europe or the USA. One of his six siblings died at age 25 with an unknown progressive lung ailment.

Physical examination was notable for a thin male; BP was 110/75 mmHg, HR was 104 beats/min, respiratory rate was 22 breaths/min, oxygen saturation 96% at rest; chest with diminished breath sounds and a prolonged expiratory phase, slightly elevated jugular venous pressure, scaphoid abdomen, no hepatomegaly, but with a trace of pedal oedema. His haematocrit was 45% and other laboratory tests were normal.

Chest radiograph shows flat diaphragm with increased radiolucency at the lung bases.

Lung function tests	Measured	Predicted (%)
FEV$_1$ (L)	0.80	20
FVC (L)	3.0	60
FEV$_1$/FVC	0.27	33
TLC (L)	8.1	120
D_LCO (mL/min per mmHg)	14	45

Questions

1 What would you expect the patient's FRC and residual volume (RV) to be?

2 Why is the cardiac point of maximal impulse (PMI) shifted to the midline?

3 Why is the FVC low?

4 Why is the D_LCO low?

5 What will happen to the patient's oxygenation with exercise? Why?

6 Why is the patient's jugular venous pressure elevated?

7 What are the most likely diagnosis and pathophysiology of his disease?

Case 4

Two 60-year-old patients are being evaluated for dyspnoea. On examination, both patients have an oxygen saturation of 88%, small lung volumes to percussion and normal cardiac examinations. Patient A has diffuse bilateral inspiratory crackles and digital clubbing. Patient B has clear lungs and difficulty in rising from his chair and raising his hands over his head.

Lung function tests	Patient A		Patient B	
	Measured	Predicted (%)	Measured	Predicted (%)
FEV$_1$ (L)	1.1	26	1.1	26
FVC (L)	1.3	26	1.3	26
FEV$_1$/FVC	0.80	100	0.80	100
TLC (L)	3.0	43	3.8	54
FRC (L)	2.0	54	3.1	87
RV (L)	1.7	65	2.5	120
D_LCO (mL/min per mmHg)	18	50	36	100

Questions

1 What patterns of abnormalities do these patients exhibit?

2 Based on the lung function results, what is the most likely pathophysiology explaining each patient's symptoms?

3 What is the likely explanation for the differences in FRC and RV between the two patients?

4 What is the differential diagnosis for Patient A?

5 What is the differential diagnosis for Patient B?

6 Both patients have hypoxaemia. Which patient is more likely to have hypercapnia?

Case 5

A 31-year-old married Vietnamese woman presented to the Accident and Emergency department following an episode of haemoptysis in which she had expectorated 250 mL fresh red blood. Nasopharyngeal examination by the ENT surgeons was normal, and a chest radiograph (Fig. 45) in the Accident and Emergency department was unhelpful, although bronchial wall thickening was noted behind the heart (arrow). There was no further bleeding, and she was discharged with an outpatient

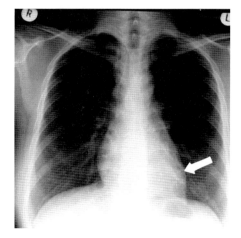

Figure 45 Chest radiograph.

appointment. Over the next few days, she continued to expectorate small clots of blood mixed with discoloured phlegm.

At her outpatient appointment, she reported a 10-year history of recurrent, intermittent haemoptysis in which she had expectorated small quantities of fresh red blood, sometimes mixed with bronchial secretions. She had been investigated by several doctors, but chest radiographs were normal, and she had been reassured that the bleeding was from the upper respiratory tract. For the 6 months before her presentation to the Accident and Emergency department, she had coughed up small quantities of blood every 2–3 weeks (<50 mL), but there was no associated fever, wheeze or breathlessness on these occasions. Two weeks before presentation to the Accident and Emergency department, she developed a cough productive of purulent sputum and night-time sweating. As a child, she had suffered with whooping cough, but there was no other past medical history of serious chest illness or tuberculosis. She is a non-smoker.

Examination was normal. She did not have finger clubbing, anaemia, cyanosis or lymphadenopathy. Chest examination was unremarkable. The breath sounds were vesicular, and there were no crackles or wheezes. Routine blood tests, including an erythrocyte sedimentation rate (ESR) and C-reactive protein and sputum microbiology including examination for tuberculosis, were normal. The grade 1 Heaf test was consistent with immunity to tuberculosis.

Questions

1 *What are the most common causes of haemoptysis, and from which circulation does bleeding occur?*
2 *Is haemoptysis life-threatening, and how is the severity of bleeding classified?*
3 *What are the clinical features that may help establish the diagnosis? What is the most likely cause in this case?*
4 *What investigations would you perform to establish the diagnosis in this case?*
5 *What is bronchiectasis, and what causes it?*
6 *How should a large haemoptysis be managed?*

Case 6

Three men have been admitted with progressive breathlessness and all have an initial arterial PaO_2 of 6.6 kPa when breathing air. The first patient is grossly obese and is complaining of a sore throat and an upper respiratory tract infection but has a normal chest CXR. Investigation has excluded pulmonary embolism. The second patient with non-specific interstitial pneumonitis has a reduced gas transfer (i.e. mainly diffusion defect), is on treatment with steroids and has developed a mild lower respiratory tract infection. The third patient has a true right to left shunt due to a longstanding atrial septal defect, and apart from a slightly enlarged heart has a normal CXR. Each patient is to be treated with oxygen.

Questions

1 *Why is each patient hypoxaemic and what will happen when the FiO_2 is raised to 1.0 (i.e. 100% oxygen therapy)? Precise answers cannot be calculated but assume reasonable values for unknown data.*
2 *How will you ensure improved oxygenation in each patient?*

Case 7

The wife and daughter of a patient you are treating for lung cancer are concerned about their risk of developing cancer. The wife has smoked for 40 years and has a 40-pack/year history but is keen to stop. The daughter has never smoked but has had lifelong passive cigarette-smoke exposure.

Questions

1 *What are the risks associated with cigarette smoking?*
2 *Why is smoking addictive?*
3 *How would you advise the wife regarding smoking cessation?*
4 *Following smoking cessation what is the risk of developing cancer?*
5 *What are the effects of passive smoking on children?*

Case 8

James is a 1.93 m tall basketball player who is 22 years old and very fit. He has previously been in excellent health. After a game, he suddenly develops a severe, sharp stabbing pain in his upper right chest and pectoral regions, and begins to feel out of breath; both his heart and respiratory rates increase dramatically. His coach immediately takes him to hospital. James tells you that he suffered no major collisions or injuries during the game, and on examination you find no bruising. You suspect a primary spontaneous pneumothorax (PSP).

Questions:

1 *What brings you to suspect PSP?*
2 *How do you confirm your diagnosis?*
3 *What causes PSP, and is it likely to happen to James again?*
4 *What treatment would you prescribe?*
5 *You advise him neither to play another game for at least some months nor to climb Mount Kilimanjaro, which he had intended to do for charity. Why?*

Case studies: answers

Case 1: Pulmonary emboli

1 Pulmonary embolism can be asymptomatic or present with a variety of different symptoms and signs including sudden death. Breathlessness and pain, which is typically pleuritic, are the most common symptoms followed by cough. Haemoptysis is relatively uncommon occurring in only about one in six patients. Other presentations and symptoms include hypotension and syncope, wheezing, and sudden onset of atrial fibrillation. Symptoms and signs of a deep venous thrombosis (DVT), such as swelling and pain in the calf, may also be present, but they are often absent. Both these patients have had recent orthopaedic surgery and are in a high-risk group for DVT and pulmonary embolus. In this context, sudden onset of breathlessness and/or pleuritic pain makes pulmonary embolism a serious possibility. In patients without a history of recent surgery or fracture presenting in an Accident and Emergency department with recent onset of breathlessness or pleuritic pain, pulmonary embolus would be a less likely explanation for these symptoms but still a real possibility even in those with no other recognized risk factors (see Answer 3).

2 Either of these oxygen saturations is entirely compatible with the diagnosis of pulmonary embolus. A low P_aO_2 and arterial oxygen saturation are common especially with the larger, more proximally lodged emboli, whereas oxygen saturation may be normal with smaller emboli that lodge more peripherally.

3 No, with a moderately increased physiological dead-space hypoxia can be avoided if the subject increases respiratory rate and/or tidal volume sufficiently to compensate for the increased dead-space ventilation, restoring alveolar ventilation to its previous level. However, pulmonary embolism leads to other problems such as reduced surfactant production, areas of atelectasis and increased ventilation–perfusion mismatching. The effects of ventilation–perfusion mismatching may be made worse by decreased mixed venous oxygen content, resulting from a reduced cardiac output. As a result, hypoxia and an increased A–a P_O_2 gradient are common with pulmonary emboli. As expected with ventilation–perfusion mismatching, P_aCO_2 is usually reduced.

4 Other risk factors may be revealed. These include pregnancy, oestrogen therapy, cancer, malignancy, chemotherapy, previous DVT, myocardial infarction, inflammatory bowel disease, immobilization or recent long distance travel. A previous or family history of venous thrombosis will suggest an inherited problem with the coagulation system such as factor V Leiden. On examination a raised jugular venous pressure and/or a pleural rub would increase suspicion.

5 D-dimers are fibrin degradation products. They are not specific to pulmonary embolus or DVT but may be raised in sepsis, trauma (including surgery) and malignancy so false-positives are common. With the most sensitive assays, false-negatives are less common but may occur with small peripheral emboli. Following a pulmonary embolus, they remain elevated for about 6 days following the onset of symptoms. In the clinical context of low probability of pulmonary embolus, negative D-dimers can be the end of the investigation. If D-dimers are positive or clinical probability high then further investigation is likely to be appropriate.

Small peripheral emboli may also be missed by other techniques such as computed tomography pulmonary angiogram (CTPA). They tend to cause pleuritic pain but less breathlessness and haemodynamic disturbance than larger emboli, which lodge in more proximal pulmonary arteries. There is some controversy about whether failing to detect such emboli matters. They are likely to clear without treatment but on the other hand they may herald further, more significant emboli.

6 Both the chest X-ray (CXR) and the electrocardiogram (ECG) may show abnormalities, but none of the abnormalities are specific to pulmonary emboli. In the presence of a pulmonary embolus, the X-ray may be normal initially but abnormalities such as areas of atelectasis, parenchymal densities and pleural effusions often develop over the first day or so. Pleural effusions are usually small, often bloody and resolve over a few days. An increasing pleural effusion suggests another cause for the symptoms or recurrent emboli. The ECG may be completely normal or show non-specific changes. Other changes that may be found are associated with right ventricular strain such as the S1, Q3, T3 pattern (prominent S wave in lead I, Q wave and inverted T in lead III), right axis deviation, dominant R wave in lead V1, inverted T waves in leads V1–V3 and right bundle-branch block.

Probably the most important role of the CXR and ECG is to reveal alternative causes of symptoms such as dyspnoea and chest pain, such as pneumothorax or myocardial infarction.

7 Diagnosing pulmonary emboli is difficult and as yet there is no single test that is highly sensitive, highly specific, non-invasive, readily available and suitable for all situations. Various algorithms and investigation strategies have been proposed that take into account risk factors and the clinical situation, but this still remains a difficult area with problems of both under- and overdiagnosis. Radionuclide ventilation–perfusion scans, spiral/helical computed tomography (CTPA) and pulmonary angiograms – all have advantages and disadvantages, which are discussed in Chapter 28. Demonstrating a DVT using Doppler imaging or venography is helpful, both because it greatly increases the likelihood that pulmonary symptoms are embolic in origin and also because the treatment is the same for both.

8 Anticoagulation with heparin and then warfarin for 6 months is the standard treatment for proven pulmonary emboli (see Chapter 28), but for Elizabeth and Alice this option is complicated by their recent surgery, which would increase the risk of haemorrhagic complications. An inferior vena cava filter is an alternative and may be necessary to prevent further fatal emboli. This is a further reason why vigorous prophylaxis (see Chapter 28) is essential in high-risk patients. Thrombolysis is sometimes considered in large emboli with haemodynamic effects but would be contraindicated here by the recent surgery.

Case 2: Asthma

1 For males, peak flow should be no more than 100 L/min below the predicted; Tom's peak flow is therefore within the normal range for his age and size. The most useful value to compare it with would be his own best peak flow rate.

2 All of these should be normal. Asthma, especially in the young, is reversible, and between attacks patients usually have normal airway resistance, compliance, lung volumes and blood gases. Peak flow and auscultation (but see note in Answer 9) suggest little evidence of airway obstruction today.

3 Simple observations that can be made in these circumstances are as follow:

- How breathless is he? Inability to talk in complete sentences is an indication of a severe attack.
- Respiratory rate (>25 breaths/min suggests a severe attack).
- Cyanosis (very severe attack).
- Pulse rate (>110 beats/min suggests a severe attack).
- If he has his peak flow meter with him, a value of more than 50% of his best or predicted suggests severe attack.

Even in the absence of the above signs of a severe attack, it is important to monitor the response to treatment to ensure that improvement rather than deterioration is occurring. He should use a short-acting β_2-adrenoreceptor agonist (salbutamol), which relaxes bronchial smooth muscle (see Chapter 25).

4 He now has definite bronchoconstriction; we would expect both peak flow and FEV_1/FVC to be reduced. In this mild attack, he would probably be able to exhale completely, so functional residual capacity (FRC) is likely to be normal. There is at present no reason why lung compliance should be altered. Although he will be working harder than normal, he should be achieving a normal alveolar ventilation and his blood gases should be normal. A reduced arterial P_{CO_2} may be caused by anxiety and consequent hyperventilation.

5 Expiratory rhonchi (musical sounds caused by vibration of the sides of collapsing airways).

6 The broken sentences, use of accessory muscles, high heart and respiratory rate are all important. The peak flow is only about 40% of his best value.

7 This is clearly a severe asthma attack, and airway resistance would be greatly increased. It is likely that air trapping would occur, as initially expiration is affected more than inspiration. As expiration is slowed, the subject may be forced to breathe in before the last breath has been fully exhaled, or air may be trapped behind collapsed airways. This would lead to a raised FRC. The volume–pressure curve flattens as total lung capacity (TLC) is approached (i.e. compliance is reduced). Consequently, with this severity of attack, the work of breathing is increased not only because of increased work against airway resistance, but also because of increased elastic resistance. In addition, with increased FRC, the inspiratory muscles may not be at their optimum working length and hence efficiency is impaired. Some ventilation–perfusion mismatching would be expected, as bronchoconstriction and inflammation will result in underventilation of some regions, and with the resulting shunt effect there is likely to be some degree of arterial hypoxia. Increased total ventilation will usually lower the P_{CO_2}, resulting in a final blood gas picture of low P_{O_2} and low P_{CO_2}.

8 The cyanosis indicates severe hypoxia, and is probably responsible for his confused mental state. The inability to talk and produce a peak flow reading is also signs of life-threatening asthma. The disappearance of rhonchi is consistent with very poor air movement. Rhonchi are a characteristic feature of airway obstruction, but they are not a reliable indicator of severity. In life-threatening asthma, the normal vesicular breath sounds are also absent. A silent chest in an asthma attack is an ominous sign.

9 The low P_aO_2 is caused by ventilation–perfusion mismatching. Hypoxia is what kills in severe asthma, so it is appropriate to give high inspired oxygen, which should significantly raise alveolar oxygen tension in poorly ventilated regions of his lung, and so improve arterial oxygenation. In this patient, there is no need to worry about ventilatory drive, so as high as possible is the correct emergency treatment. With a face mask, the maximum achievable is approximately 60%. Although a

P_{CO_2} of 5.5 kPa would usually be considered 'normal', in the presence of severe hypoxia it should be regarded as worrying. With this degree of hypoxia, the drive to breathing should be increased, with increased ventilation and low P_{CO_2}. Here, the failure to raise ventilation appropriately is likely to indicate exhaustion. The patient may deteriorate rapidly – a further fall in ventilation will worsen hypoxia, and this may be fatal. In the presence of significant hypoxia, a 'normal' or high arterial P_{CO_2} should be regarded as a serious finding.

Case 3: Severe breathlessness

1 The obstructive ventilatory defect (low ratio of FEV_1/FVC) coupled with a reduced diffusing capacity for carbon monoxide would suggest emphysema. Emphysema is characterized by a reduction in lung elastic recoil, increased lung compliance and floppy airways. Therefore, FRC and residual volume (RV) are both likely to be elevated.

2 The hyperinflation of the lung and the increase in FRC pull the apex of the heart caudally and to the middle. This can be seen radiographically as a small midline heart. The ECG will show low voltage due to the increased amount of air between the heart and the chest wall, with an axis close to $90°$. For a similar reason, the apex beat may be quiet.

3 The forced vital capacity (FVC) is low because the RV is high. Airways close prematurely in emphysema, which increases RV. Furthermore, because of the marked decrease in maximal expiratory flow rate due to the decreased lung elastic recoil, patients' spirometry traces may not plateau, indicating that the lung was still emptying at very low flow rates when the FVC manoeuvre was terminated.

4 Diffusing capacity is influenced by the alveolar–capillary surface area for gas exchange. Emphysema is characterized by a loss of the alveolar–capillary units that are utilized for diffusion. There need not be a defect in transfer of gas from the alveolus to the capillary to reduce the D_LCO; a reduction in surface area is adequate to cause abnormality.

5 With exercise, the patient's oxygen saturation will fall because of the diffusion defect. With this magnitude of diffusion defect, the red cells have adequate time to equilibrate with alveolar oxygen as they traverse the alveolar–capillary membrane. However, during exercise, when cardiac output rises, red cells traverse the alveolar–capillary membrane at rest more quickly and do not equilibrate with alveolar oxygen tension at the end-capillary segment. This results in deoxygenated blood entering the systemic circulation when cardiac output is increased. This exercise-induced desaturation will be accentuated when alveolar oxygen is reduced, such as at high altitude. The threshold for significant oxygen desaturation with exercise is approximately $D_LCO < 50\%$ predicted.

6 The patient probably has a component of pulmonary hypertension due to the emphysema. The loss of capillary units raises pulmonary vascular resistance and increases right heart work. Any degree of hypoxaemia during exercise will exacerbate the pulmonary hypertension by superimposing hypoxic pulmonary vasoconstriction on the already increased resistance.

7 The presence of early onset emphysema, the family history and the history of cigarette smoking make the diagnosis of α_1-antitrypsin (AAT) deficiency most likely. He probably has the homozygous ZZ genotype that causes a marked reduction of AAT levels to less than 15% normal. The radiograph is consistent with panacinar emphysema and alveolar destruction predominantly at the bases. The lung destruction is due to release of proteolytic enzymes from neutrophils and other inflammatory cells in response to environmental stimuli. These enzymes are normally neutralized by the antiproteases in the lung to prevent lung destruction in the presence of mild inflammatory stimuli. In AAT deficiency, the proteases are not neutralized, and induce panacinar emphysema under 'normal' circumstances. Cigarette smoking induces a neutrophilic response in the lung that accelerates the decline of lung function in AAT deficiency. Intravenous replacement of AAT in patients with reduced lung function may slow the decline in FEV_1.

Case 4: Restrictive ventilatory defect

1 Both patients have restrictive ventilatory defects based on the reduced TLC. FEV_1 and FVC are reduced proportionally, so the FEV_1/FVC is normal; therefore, there is no obstructive ventilatory defect. Patient A has reduced $D_L CO$, signifying a gas transfer defect.

2 Restrictive ventilatory defects may be due to stiff lungs, stiff chest wall or weak respiratory muscles. Diseases causing stiff lungs will reduce all lung volumes/capacities simultaneously, including TLC, FRC and RV. Most parenchymal lung diseases will also cause a reduced $D_L CO$, whereas chest wall disease and respiratory muscle disease will not. An increased RV is also not compatible with stiff lungs. Thus, Patient A seems to have a problem with stiff lungs. The relatively normal FRC and $D_L CO$ in Patient B suggest that the lungs and chest wall are normal. Either a stiff chest wall or weak muscles may cause an increased RV. Patient B's lung function and difficulty in rising out of a chair and raising his arms suggest a muscle disease. Diseases causing weak respiratory muscles will reduce TLC, because the patient cannot inspire deeply.

3 The FRC is determined by the balance between the inward pull of the lung elastic recoil pressure and the outward pull of the chest wall. Therefore, FRC will be reduced either if the net lung recoil pressure increases (due to stiff, low-compliance lungs) or if the net outward pull of the chest wall decreases (e.g. when scarring of the chest wall produces an added inward recoiling force). Since FRC is determined by the balance between two opposing static forces, respiratory muscle weakness should not influence FRC. However, in clinical practice, patients with respiratory muscle weakness often have a slightly reduced FRC. The mechanism for this finding is probably related to the lack of deep breaths or sighs causing microatelectasis that will increase lung recoil and decrease compliance.

RV is the amount of gas remaining in the lung at the end of maximal expiration. In adults, RV is determined by airway collapse at low lung volumes. However, this presupposes adequate expiratory muscle strength to actively lower lung volume below FRC (which can be reached from TLC passively). Patient A has normal muscle strength and airways that resist collapse due to the parenchymal lung disease, resulting in a reduced RV. Patient B has weak expiratory muscles, resulting in an elevated RV.

4 The differential diagnosis is long and includes the disorders discussed in Chapter 30. Briefly, these would include occupational/environmental disorders, connective tissue/autoimmune diseases, drug/treatment-induced diseases, primary lung disorders or idiopathic disorders. Idiopathic pulmonary fibrosis or cryptogenic fibrosing alveolitis is likely in a 60-year-old with lung crackles, clubbing, no significant past history, no signs or symptoms of extrapulmonary disease and the lung function shown for Patient A.

5 Respiratory muscle weakness may be due to a variety of neuromuscular diseases that can involve the spinal cord, motor nerves, neuromuscular junction or skeletal muscles:

- Spinal cord: tumour, syringomyelia, polio, amyotrophic lateral sclerosis, tetanus
- Motor nerves: brachial/phrenic nerve neuritis, trauma.

- Neuromuscular junction: myasthenia gravis, botulism, organophosphate poisoning
- Skeletal muscle: muscular dystrophy, myositis, mitochondrial disease, myopathy (nutritional, drug, metabolic, inherited)

6 Hypoxaemia in interstitial lung diseases is usually due to ventilation–perfusion mismatching. Patient A likely has hypocapnia because patients with interstitial lung disease tend to hyperventilate in response to stiff lungs and hypoxia. This will lower arterial carbon dioxide tension. In contrast, Patient B likely has hypoxaemia due to alveolar hypoventilation, and is therefore hypercapnic. Patient B is also more likely to develop acute respiratory failure with the limited ventilatory reserve due to the muscle weakness.

Case 5: Haemoptysis

1 The table below illustrates that most cases of haemoptysis are due to infection ($\sim$80%) – including tuberculosis, pneumonia, lung abscess and bronchiectasis. Only a minority are due to malignancy ($\sim$20%). Pulmonary embolism and trauma are other potentially important causes. The bronchial (rather than the pulmonary) circulation is the usual source of bleeding.

2 Approximately 35–40% of cases of haemoptysis are classified as trivial (flecks of blood in sputum), 45–50% as moderate ($<$500 mL or 0.5–2 cups daily) and only 10–20% as massive ($>$500 mL or more than 2 cups of blood daily). Mortality is directly related to the rate and volume of blood loss and the underlying pathology. In patients expectorating more than 500 mL of blood within a 4-hour period, the mortality is approximately 70%, compared with 5% in patients expectorating the same quantity over 16–48 hours. Death results from asphyxia, caused by flooding of the alveoli and only rarely from circulatory collapse.

3 A good history is essential, and may indicate the cause of haemoptysis. The characteristic clinical picture of diseases such as tuberculosis, bronchiectasis and bronchogenic carcinoma may direct subsequent investigation and management. Chest examination may reveal localized crepitations or consolidation, but widespread soiling of the tracheobronchial tree with blood (due to coughing) often results in diffuse clinical signs. Examination of expectorated blood may provide clues. Food particles suggest the possibility of haematemesis, but blood in the nasogastric aspirate does not differentiate between haematemesis and haemoptysis, as coughed-up blood is often swallowed. Purulent material in the sputum may indicate bronchiectasis or a lung abscess. Associated haematuria raises the possibility of an alveolar haemorrhage syndrome. In this case, the age of the patient, the long history of minor haemoptysis and the symptoms of purulent sputum and night-time fever suggest a diagnosis of **bronchiectasis**, although other potential causes include recurrent pulmonary emboli, vasculitis and a benign adenoma.

Infective ($\sim$80%)	Malignant ($\sim$20%)	Other
Tuberculosis	Lung cancer	Pulmonary infarction
Pneumonia	Metastatic cancer	Adenoma
Lung abscess	Lymphoma	Traumatic
Bronchiectasis		Alveolar haemorrhage
Aspergillus		Vasculitis

4 Routine blood tests (white cell count raised in infection), including erythrocyte sedimentation rate (ESR) (raised in vasculitis) and C-reactive protein (raised in infection). Specialist blood tests (D-dimers

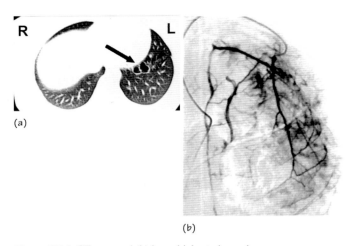

(a)

(b)

Figure 46(a) CT scan and (b) bronchial arteriography.

for pulmonary emboli, *Aspergillus* precipitans, vasculitis screen) may be required. Sputum microbiology may isolate infective organisms (pneumonia, abscess, *Aspergillus*) or acid-fast bacilli (tuberculosis). A screening Heaf test may detect tuberculosis. Chest radiography should be obtained in all patients. It may provide important diagnostic information including evidence of a mass, cavity or abscess. CT scans with contrast may detect the site of bleeding, tumours, vascular malformations and other structural abnormalities. In this case, the CT scan demonstrated a grossly dilated bronchus (>10 mm) consistent with bronchiectasis in the anteromedial segment of the left lower lobe (Fig. 46a). Bronchoscopy is often required to detect endobronchial lesions and inhaled objects (e.g. tooth). Combinations of bronchoscopy and CT scanning have the highest diagnostic yield. Bronchial arteriography may be required to detect the site of bleeding (Fig. 46b).

5 Bronchiectasis is described in Chapter 34.

6 The key aspects of management of massive haemoptysis are to maintain a patent airway and oxygenation (oxygen therapy). Asphyxia (not bleeding) is the greatest immediate risk to the patient. Promote drainage of blood and prevent alveolar 'soiling' by positioning the patient slightly head down in the lateral decubitus position, with the 'presumed' bleeding side down. Determine the cause, site and severity of the bleeding (as above): haematemesis and upper airways bleeding (e.g. nose) may be confused with haemoptysis. Treatment of the underlying cause is essential if the haemoptysis is to be controlled (antibiotics for pneumonia or a lung abscess). Avoid excessive chest manipulation, including physiotherapy, as this may increase or restart bleeding. Cough suppression with codeine 30–60 mg every 6 hours may be helpful. Institute appropriate antibiotics and bronchodilators.

Immediate control of haemoptysis is achieved at bronchoscopy by directing boluses of iced saline with epinephrine (10 mL; 1:10 000 dilution) at the bleeding site.

Bronchial angiography and **embolization** are the established therapeutic techniques for the initial control of haemoptysis. This procedure is initially successful in 70–100% of cases. The best results are described in patients with dilated bronchial arteries (e.g. bronchiectasis). Rebleeding often occurs (~40%), and infarction of the anterior spinal artery with paraplegia is reported (~5%). Most studies agree that surgical therapy is associated with the best long-term outcomes for isolated lesions. Primary medical management may be mandatory because bleeding cannot be localized (widespread *Aspergillus* infection) or is not amenable to surgical resection of a

pulmonary segment. In other patients, surgery will be contraindicated because of end-stage lung disease (FEV_1 <40% predicted), poor cardiac reserve, unresectable cancer or severe bleeding diathesis.

Final diagnosis: bronchiectasis of the anteromedial segment of the left lower lobe.

Case 6: Oxygenation and oxygen therapy
Patient 1

1 This patient has a mild upper respiratory tract infection and no significant low respiratory tract pathology. However, he is probably hypoventilating due to gross obesity restricting normal respiratory movement. Assuming his gas transfer and V/Q matching are normal, his P_aCO_2 can be calculated from the alveolar gas equation (Chapter 14):

$$P_AO_2 = P_IO_2 - \frac{P_aCO_2}{R}$$

where $P_AO_2 \approx P_aO_2 = 6.6$ kPa (as measured); $P_IO_2 = F_IO_2 \times$ (barometric − water vapour pressure) $= 0.21 \times (101 - 6.2) = 19.9$ kPa breathing air, and R, the respiratory quotient, is ~0.8. Thus, $P_aCO_2 = 10.6$ kPa and if the arterial blood gas measurement confirms this, the patient has type 2 respiratory failure (Chapter 23). If the measured P_aCO_2 was much lower, it would suggest the assumptions were wrong and that another mechanism was causing or contributing to his respiratory failure.

When the patient is given 100% O_2 (F_IO_2 1.0):

$$P_IO_2 = F_IO_2 \times \text{(barometric − water vapour pressure)}$$
$$= 1 \times (101 - 6.2) = 95 \text{ kPa}$$

So:

$$P_aO_2 \approx P_AO_2 = 95 - \frac{10.6}{0.8} = 82 \text{ kPa}$$

2 In some patients with chronic type 2 respiratory failure hypoxia drives ventilation rather than P_aCO_2. As the patient's P_aO_2 rises when he is given 100% O_2, the drive to breath decreases, and this can lead to a further increase in P_aCO_2, progressive respiratory acidosis, confusion, coma and death. Consequently, this patient should be managed with low-dose (24–28%) O_2 therapy aiming for a saturation of 88–92% and regular measurement of arterial blood gases (Chapters 23 and 43). In this patient optimal treatment to improve oxygenation and reduce CO_2 retention would be non-invasive ventilation, which would improve ventilation and alveolar gas exchange (Chapter 42).

Patient 2

1 This patient has a diffusion defect due to the interstitial lung disease (ILD, Chapter 30) although usually there is a significant contribution of ventilation/perfusion (V/Q) mismatch due to the hypoxaemia. His P_AO_2 is thus greater than his P_aO_2. Arterial blood gas (ABG) shows his P_aCO_2 is low (4 kPa). The substantial increase in P_AO_2 when this patient is given 100% oxygen ($F_IO_2 = 1$) will more than overcome the partial diffusion defect associated with the ILD, and if this were a pure diffusion defect the P_aO_2 could approach 90 kPa.

$$P_AO_2 = 95 - \frac{4}{0.8} = 90 \text{ kPa}$$

Even allowing for a wider than normal range of V/Q ratios in this patient, there would still be a substantial increase in P_aO_2 on 100% oxygen.

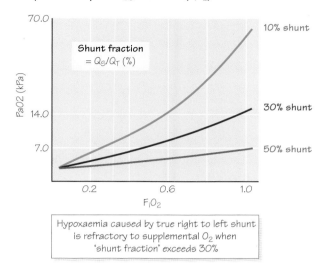

Effect of true shunt (Q_S/Q_T) on the arterial oxygen tension (P_aO_2) response to inspired oxygen fraction (F_iO_2)

Hypoxaemia caused by true right to left shunt is refractory to supplemental O_2 when 'shunt fraction' exceeds 30%

Figure 47

2 In this patient simply increasing the inspired oxygen concentration ($F_iO_2 \sim 0.4$–0.6) will correct the hypoxaemia. This patient probably has **type 1 respiratory failure** (Chapter 23) because CO_2 diffuses 20 times better than O_2 and consequently the diffusion defect does not impair CO_2 clearance. The hypoxaemia will cause hyperventilation, and the associated increase in minute ventilation ensures a low P_aCO_2 ($\propto$ 1/alveolar ventilation). Consequently, there is little risk of hypercapnia during the use of high O_2 concentrations in this patient.

Patient 3

1 This patient is hypoxaemic due true right-to-left shunting causing admixture of venous blood to systemic arterial blood (Chapter 13). As in the second case, the P_AO_2 will be 90 kPa with an F_iO_2 of 1.0. However, the saturation is already 100% in oxygenated blood passing through the lungs, and O_2 content will not be substantially increased by the high P_AO_2 apart from the small quantity of O_2 dissolved in blood (90 $\times$ 0.023 mL; Chapter 8). The blood shunted from right to left through the atrial septal defect remains unaffected by the increased P_AO_2 and acts as venous admixture lowering oxygenation in the systemic circulation. Consequently, an F_iO_2 of 1.0 only fractionally increases systemic P_aO_2 perhaps to ~ 7.5 kPa in this case.

2 Only Patient 3 will not show a substantial increase in P_aO_2 when given 100% O_2. In this case oxygenation will only be improved by decreasing the shunt fraction and reducing left-sided venous admixture. Figure 47 illustrates the effect of true shunt on the response to increasing F_iO_2.

Case 7: Smoking cessation

1 Smoking accounts for 90% of lung cancer cases and approximately 30% of all cancer deaths in developed countries. Cancers of the oropharynx, nasal cavity, nasal sinuses, larynx, oesophagus, stomach, pancreas, liver, urinary tract, uterine cervix and myeloid leukaemia are all associated with smoking. In the UK in 2005, 46 000 cancer deaths were attributed to smoking. Smoking also causes chronic obstructive pulmonary disease (COPD), coronary heart disease, peripheral vascular disease, stroke, pneumonia, interstitial lung disease, venous thromboembolism, diabetes, inflammatory bowel disease and peptic ulceration.

The relative risk of developing lung cancer in a long-term smoker compared to a lifelong non-smoker is increased by about 30-fold. The level of risk is dependent on dose (i.e. number of cigarettes/day, depth of inhalation and number of years smoked), age of onset, race (e.g. African Americans at greater risk) and pattern of smoking (i.e. a quit period reduces subsequent risk on restarting smoking).

2 High brain nicotine levels occur within 7–10 seconds of inhaling cigarette smoke. Activation of brain nicotine acetylcholine receptors (nAchR) stimulates the release of neurotransmitters (e.g. noradrenaline and serotonin), especially dopamine in the mesolimbic system (brain reward pathway), which elicits pleasure and is associated with the development of addictive behaviour. Repeated exposure to nicotine desensitises nAchR, and despite a 300% increase in the number of receptors, the response to nicotine gradually decreases and natural brain dopamine levels fall requiring increased nicotine stimulation for equivalent effect.

3 Smoking cessation is best achieved using a combination of intensive behavioural support and pharmacological therapies. Initially assess the 5As: **A**sk how much the person smokes and document pack years; **A**ssess risk of continued smoking and inform the patient; **A**dvise how to stop smoking and what help is available; **A**ssist with behavioural support or replacement therapy and **A**rrange follow-up. It is vital that the patient is well motivated and has set a quit date to stop smoking completely (i.e. 'to go cold turkey'). Slowly reducing daily cigarette consumption will not overcome the additive nature of smoking.

Quit rates with simple counselling are only 1–3%, but intensive behavioural support with telephone follow-up, web-based support and multiple interviews can achieve 20% one-year abstinence rates. **Nicotine replacement therapy** (NRT) is the most used pharmacological aid to smoking cessation. A 22 mg patch raises the baseline blood nicotine concentration to levels achieved by smoking 30 cigarettes over 24 hours. However, addition of gum or lozenges to the patch helps overcome breakthrough urges. When intensive smoking cessation support is combined with NRT, 1-year abstinence rates of 35% can be achieved. **Bupropion (Zyban)**, a dopamine uptake inhibitor, doubles the success of smoking cessation. It is started 1–2 weeks before stopping smoking and is given for 8 weeks. Combination with NRT is not always beneficial. Bupropion is contraindicated in epilepsy and pregnancy. **Varenicline (Champix)** is a new partial nAchR agonist that reduces craving and withdrawal and decreases the reward of smoking. A 12-week course is recommended and is commenced 1–2 weeks before the 'quit date'. Twelve-week quit rates in two major studies comparing vareniciline, bupropion and placebo were 45, 30 and 18%, respectively, and at 12 months were 23, 16 and 9%, respectively.

4 Smoking cessation reduces the risk of developing lung cancer by up to 90%. However, the risk of developing lung cancer is always higher than in lifelong non-smokers and is dependent on the number of cigarettes smoked, age at smoking cessation and the number of years since smoking cessation. For every year smoking cessation is postponed after 40 years old, life expectancy is reduced by 3 months. Passive smoking is associated with both morbidity and mortality. Non-smokers who live with smokers have a 24% increase in the incidence of lung cancer. The risk is 16–19% in those exposed to passive smoking in the workplace.

5 Passive smoking is harmful in children and increases respiratory disease, asthma attacks, cot deaths and middle ear infections. In the UK over 30% of children live with at least one adult smoker, and

among low-income families this increases to 57%. Smoking during pregnancy is associated with increased risk of spontaneous abortion, preterm birth, low birth weight and stillbirth. In 2005, 32% of women smoked before or during pregnancy and 17% throughout pregnancy. These figures were 48 and 29%, respectively, in lower socioeconomic groups.

Case 8: Primary spontaneous pneumothorax

1 Primary spontaneous pneumothorax (PSP) is the most common form of pneumothorax, and is most usually observed in otherwise healthy young men, particularly those over 1.9 m in height. Your suspicion is aroused because James falls into such a category, and in particular by the sudden onset of sharp pleuritic pain and breathlessness.

2 Diagnosis is confirmed by X-ray. Unless the pneumothorax is large, other clinical signs such as a hyperresonant chest may be difficult to detect.

3 PSP occurs when an apical bleb on the surface of the lung ruptures, commonly in the upper lobes. This allows air from the airways to enter the space between the visceral and parietal pleura, causing partial or complete collapse of the lung. The pleural space is normally regarded as a 'potential' space, because it is usually filled with a thin layer of fluid that provides traction between the chest wall and lungs, so that the elastic recoil of the lungs is balanced by the outward recoil of the chest wall. The pleural pressure is therefore normally negative with respect to that in the airways and atmosphere (Chapter 3). The likelihood of developing PSP is more than 20 times greater in people taller than 1.9 m. The risk increases sharply (>60%) after a second episode.

4 James is lucky in that in his case the PSP is less than 30% of lung volume. This should naturally resolve, so you prescribe analgesics for the pain and rest, and tell him to come back and see you over the next few weeks for serial chest X-rays to confirm resolution. If the PSP was more than 30% (moderate), the pneumothorax would be aspirated, and the patient prescribed oxygen and admitted overnight, with an X-ray in the morning to confirm lung re-expansion. Complete lung collapse would require a chest drain (Chapter 35).

If James were to suffer repeated PSP, consideration would have to be given to pleurodesis, where the visceral and parietal pleura fuse as a result of either insertion of bleomycin or talc into the pleural space, or surgical abrasion of the pleura.

5 Both the high exertion of a basketball game and the reduced barometric pressure and hence PO_2 at the summit of Mount Kilimanjaro would strongly stimulate breathing. This would lead to much more negative pressures in the intrapleural space, which could substantially increase the risk of another PSP.

Self-assessment questions

Choose the single **best** answer from the options for each question. Answers on page 118.

Chapter 1: Structure of the respiratory system: lungs, airways and dead space

1.1 The pulmonary nerve plexus
- (a) contains sympathetic nerves which are the main mechanism of bronchodilatation
- (b) contains parasympathetic bronchoconstrictor nerves
- (c) surrounds each lung in the visceral pleura
- (d) contain non-adrenergic non-cholinergic (NANC) nerves that travel with the intercostal nerves

1.2 The pleural space
- (a) around the left lung connects to that around the right lung so that a pneumothorax on one side usually spreads to the other
- (b) extends below the lungs as the costodiaphragmatic recess only during expiration
- (c) lies between the parietal and visceral pleura
- (d) normally contains a few hundred mL of fluid

1.3 Type II pneumocytes
- (a) make up most of the area of the alveolar epithelium
- (b) are unable to divide to produce new cells
- (c) are ciliated
- (d) are the main source of pulmonary surfactant

1.4 Alveolar dead space
- (a) is increased in someone who has a pulmonary embolus
- (b) in a normal person is about 150 mL
- (c) is normally about the same size as the physiological dead space
- (d) is increased by the presence of consolidation in lobar pneumonia

Chapter 2: The thoracic cage and respiratory muscles

2.1 Intercostal spaces
- (a) contain an intercostal nerve, intercostal vein and intercostal artery lying just above the top of the rib
- (b) contain the main expiratory muscles
- (c) are stiffened during inspiration and expiration by the contraction of the intercostal muscles
- (d) contain muscles which are too weak to maintain adequate resting ventilation if the diaphragm is paralysed

2.2 The diaphragm
- (a) has sensory innervation from the same cervical roots as the shoulder
- (b) has the oesophagus passing through it at the aortic opening
- (c) contracts upwards during expiration
- (d) is less important than the other inspiratory muscles in the newborn

2.3 Accessory inspiratory muscles include all of the following EXCEPT
- (a) the sternomastoids
- (b) serratus anterior
- (c) pectoralis major
- (d) rectus abdominis

2.4 Paradoxical breathing
- (a) will follow bilateral phrenic nerve destruction
- (b) refers to an unusual pattern of breathing in which the abdomen moves out as the chest wall is moving out in inspiration
- (c) is normal in babies
- (d) will follow a cervical cord transection at C3

Chapter 3: Pressures and volumes during normal breathing

3.1 Functional residual capacity
- (a) is the volume left in the lungs after a maximum expiration
- (b) is the sum of residual volume and tidal volume
- (c) is affected by the elastic recoil of both the lungs and chest wall but not the strength of the inspiratory or expiratory muscles
- (d) is the volume in the lungs when intrapleural pressure is about 0.5 kPa above atmospheric

3.2 Intrapleural pressure
- (a) is usually measured by putting a needle through the ribs into the intrapleural space
- (b) is negative (below atmospheric pressure) throughout the respiratory cycle during quiet breathing
- (c) is always higher than alveolar pressure at the same level
- (d) is more negative at the lung bases than the lung apices in an upright subject

3.3 From the trace produced when a subject breathes in and out of a simple water-filled spirometer, it is possible to measure
- (a) functional residual capacity
- (b) vital capacity
- (c) total lung capacity
- (d) residual volume

3.4 The predicted lung volumes for a subject
- (a) are helpful because they avoid the necessity for measuring the subject's lung volumes
- (b) are the average lung volumes for someone of the same age, weight and gender of the subject
- (c) are needed to interpret lung volumes because the range in healthy adults is very large
- (d) are needed because lung volumes vary greatly in healthy subjects from day to day

Chapter 4: Gas laws

4.1 Fractional concentration of oxygen in the air
- (a) reduces progressively with increasing altitude
- (b) multiplied by barometric pressure gives the partial pressure of oxygen in the air
- (c) is about 0.78 (= 78%) at sea level
- (d) divided by barometric pressure gives the partial pressure of oxygen in the air

4.2 Saturated water vapour pressure
- (a) falls as temperature rises
- (b) in the lungs is greater in a man on Everest than in a man at sea level
- (c) in the lungs is the normally 13 kPa (100 mmHg)
- (d) is the maximum water vapour pressure that is possible at a given temperature

4.3 A man has eaten a lunch of baked beans on toast and drunk a bottle of cola after which he goes on a hot air balloon ride. As he ascends he experiences abdominal pain. The gas law that best explains his problem is
  (a) Charles' law (V ∝ T)
  (b) Boyle's law (V ∝ 1/P)
  (c) Henry's law (concentration of a gas in a liquid ∝ partial pressure of the gas in a liquid)
  (d) Dalton's law (partial pressure of a gas in a mixture = fractional concentration of the gas × total pressure of the mixture)

4.4 When the lid was removed from the bottle of cola, bubbles formed in the liquid and rose to the surface.

The gas law that best explains his problem is
  (a) Charles' law (V ∝ T)
  (b) Boyle's law (V ∝ 1/P)
  (c) Henry's law (concentration of a gas in a liquid ∝ partial pressure of the gas in a liquid)
  (d) Dalton's law (partial pressure of a gas in a mixture = fractional concentration of the gas × total pressure of the mixture)

Chapter 5: Diffusion

5.1 Diffusion through the alveolar–capillary membrane
  (a) is slower for carbon dioxide than for oxygen because its molecular weight is higher
  (b) occurs at a rate which is proportional to the difference in concentration (mL gas per mL fluid) on either side of the membrane
  (c) is unaffected by oedema fluid in the alveolus because it is only cells that act as a barrier to diffusion
  (d) is slower for gases with low solubility in the membrane

5.2 Diffusion-limited uptake of a gas through the alveolar–capillary membrane
  (a) occurs when the gas in the alveolus reaches equilibrium with gas in the pulmonary capillary blood early in the journey through the pulmonary capillary
  (b) applies to the uptake of nitrous oxide (N_2O)
  (c) would mean that the rate of uptake of the gas would be improved if the area of the alveolar–capillary membrane increased
  (d) applies to oxygen uptake in a healthy person at sea level

5.3 Carbon monoxide (CO) diffusing capacity (transfer factor)
  (a) cannot be measured in patients with respiratory disease because carbon monoxide is too toxic
  (b) equals the CO uptake from the lungs divided by the alveolar partial pressure of CO, following inhalation of a CO-containing gas mixture
  (c) is measurable because PCO rises rapidly in the pulmonary capillary to quickly equal alveolar PCO
  (d) is only affected by the thickness of the alveolar capillary membrane

5.4 One condition that does NOT reduce the carbon monoxide diffusing capacity (transfer factor) is
  (a) anaemia
  (b) hypoventilation
  (c) lung fibrosis
  (d) emphysema

Chapter 6: Lung mechanics: elastic forces

6.1 When producing a pressure–volume loop for the measurement of static lung compliance

  (a) intrapleural pressure is usually assessed using a cannula passed between the ribs into the intrapleural space
  (b) lung compliance is calculated as volume/intrapleural pressure at functional residual capacity
  (c) the pressure–volume relationship is the same during inspiration and expiration
  (d) measurements of volume and intrapleural pressure are taken as the subject holds his breath because then alveolar pressure is zero

6.2 Surfactant
  (a) is a mixture of carbohydrates and proteins
  (b) is produced by type 1 alveolar cells
  (c) stores are often exhausted in babies who are born after the normal 40 weeks of pregnancy, giving rise to respiratory distress syndrome
  (d) is more effective at lowering the surface tension as the alveoli and airways get smaller in expiration

6.3 Low static lung compliance
  (a) can often be deduced from measurements of lung volumes and from forced expiratory spirograms, without a formal measurement of lung compliance
  (b) occurs in patients with emphysema
  (c) occurs in asthma
  (d) is associated with decreased recoil

6.4 Dynamic pressure–volume (P–V) loops differ from static pressure–volume loops in that
  (a) dynamic P–V loops cannot be used to assess lung compliance
  (b) for dynamic P–V loops the subject asked to breathe in and out as hard and fast as possible
  (c) dynamic P–V loops are 'fatter' because while air is moving, larger intrapleural pressure changes are needed to overcome airway resistance in addition to elastic resistance
  (d) dynamic P–V loops are easier to obtain because oesophageal pressure is not needed

Chapter 7: Lung mechanics: airway resistance

7.1 Airway resistance in the human lung is
  (a) greatest in the generation of distal bronchioles in healthy people because these airways have the smallest radii
  (b) not increased during a forced expiration in a healthy subject
  (c) inversely proportional to the radius in a given airway
  (d) decreased when breathing through the mouth

7.2 Airway smooth muscle constriction is
  (a) reduced by reflex stimulation of sympathetic nerves to airway smooth muscle
  (b) is inhibited when pulmonary stretch receptor reflexes are activated
  (c) increases when irritant receptors release histamine
  (d) increased by stress via the action on epinephrine (adrenaline) on airway smooth muscle

7.3 During a forced expiration
  (a) peak expiratory flow is not much affected by the effort the subject uses
  (b) flow towards the end of a breath from total lung capacity to residual volume is not much affected by the effort the subject uses
  (c) dynamic compression of airways is mostly a problem during forced inspiration

    (d) peak expiratory flow is not much affected by the initial lung volume

7.4 Airway resistance
    (a) is normal in patients with pure emphysema
    (b) can be assumed to be present if the peak expiratory flow is reduced
    (c) can assumed to be present if the forced expiratory ration (FER) is reduced
    (d) is always abnormal in a patient with asthma

Chapter 8: Carriage of oxygen
8.1 Haemoglobin
    (a) is composed of four identical subunits
    (b) has iron at the centre of haem groups which must be in the ferrous form to bind O_2
    (c) binding of oxygen is reduced in the presence of high P_{CO_2} because CO_2 and O_2 compete for the same binding sites on haemoglobin
    (d) variants (such as fetal haemoglobin) often differ from normal adult haemoglobin in the precise structure of the haem group

8.2 In an anaemic patient
    (a) arterial PO_2 is reduced
    (b) arterial oxygen saturation is reduced
    (c) resting oxygen extraction is increased
    (d) resting mixed venous PO_2 is reduced

8.3 A low P_{50}
    (a) means that the affinity of haemoglobin for oxygen is reduced
    (b) may occur in a patient with a fever
    (c) normally occurs as blood passes through tissue capillaries
    (d) occurs in the presence of fetal haemoglobin

8.4 Replacing inspired air with a gas mixture contains 60% oxygen
    (a) causes a large increase in arterial PO_2 and a small increase in oxygen content in a healthy person at sea level
    (b) causes a large increase in oxygen content with little increase in oxygen saturation in a healthy person at high altitude
    (c) would greatly reduce the exercise intolerance of a patient with severe anaemia
    (d) would greatly reduce the oxygen delivery problems of a patient in circulatory shock

Chapter 9: Carriage of carbon dioxide
9.1 CO_2 is transported in mixed venous blood as approximately
    (a) 70% bicarbonate, 29% carbamino compounds, <1% dissolved
    (b) 60% bicarbonate, 20% carbamino compounds, 20% dissolved
    (c) 60% bicarbonate, 30% carbamino compounds, 10% dissolved
    (d) 50% bicarbonate, 35% carbamino compounds, 15% dissolved

9.2 Decreased pH within the red blood cell
    (a) promotes O_2 binding to haemoglobin
    (b) causes formation of carbamino compounds
    (c) impairs O_2 delivery to tissues
    (d) is limited by haemoglobin

9.3 The Haldane effect states that
    (a) an increase in P_{CO_2} shifts the O_2 dissociation curve to the left
    (b) for any given P_{CO_2} more CO_2 is carried by oxygenated blood
    (c) for any given P_{CO_2} less CO_2 is carried by oxygenated blood
    (d) an increase in P_{CO_2} reduces the amount of haemoglobin in the red cell

9.4 Hyperventilation
    (a) occurs during exercise

    (b) causes acidosis
    (c) is defined by a P_{aCO_2} <5.9 kPa
    (d) can cause carpopedal spasm

Chapter 10: Control of acid–base balance
10.1 The Henderson–Hasselbalch equation
    (a) can only be applied to blood samples taken from the subject, but not in vivo
    (b) assumes that the concentration of carbonic acid is equal to the P_{CO_2}
    (c) employs the same value for pK for all weak acids
    (d) relates pH to the pK and concentrations of weak acid and conjugate base

10.2 Which of the following statements about buffers is true?
    (a) The maximal buffering capacity occurs when pH = pK.
    (b) The pH of a buffered solution remains constant no matter how much acid or base is added to the solution.
    (c) Weak acids and bases are not useful as buffers.
    (d) Proteins contribute very little to the buffering capacity of blood.

10.3 Why do CO_2 and bicarbonate provide a good buffer system for the blood?
    (a) They do not; haemoglobin is the primary buffer.
    (b) The pK of bicarbonate/carbonic acid is equal to the pH of blood.
    (c) Blood bicarbonate is at a high concentration compared to that of CO_2.
    (d) They are actively regulated by the lungs and kidneys, respectively.

10.4 An arterial blood sample from a patient has a pH of 7.25, P_{CO_2} of 6.6 kPa, and a base excess of −3. What is the mostly likely acid–base status of the patient? (hint: look at Chapter 10, panel c)
    (a) metabolic acidosis
    (b) uncompensated respiratory acidosis
    (c) respiratory acidosis combined with metabolic acidosis
    (d) compensated respiratory acidosis

Chapter 11: Control of breathing I: chemical mechanisms
11.1 Ventilation is NOT increased by
    (a) increased P_{aCO_2}
    (b) decreased arterial pH
    (c) decreased PO_2 at the central chemoreceptor
    (d) decreased CSF pH

11.2 The peripheral chemoreceptors
    (a) are located in the carotid sinus and aortic arch
    (b) are responsible for 80% of the ventilator response to increased P_{CO_2}
    (c) respond to changes in arterial pH
    (d) contain type II cells which detect hypoxia

11.3 The central chemoreceptor
    (a) response is dependent on the $[HCO_3^-]$ of the CSF
    (b) is located on the ventrolateral surface of the pons
    (c) responds to changes in arterial pH
    (d) directly responds to CO_2

11.4 The ventilatory response to increased P_{CO_2}
    (a) is decreased by metabolic acidosis
    (b) is unaffected by the PO_2 until the PO_2 falls below 6 kPa

(c) decreases in chronic hypercapnia

(d) is increased by inhibitors of carbonic anhydrase

Chapter 12: Control of breathing II: neural mechanisms

12.1 The receptors located on the bronchial walls close to the capillaries are

(a) pulmonary stretch receptors

(b) juxtapulmonary receptors

(c) irritant receptors

(d) proprioceptors

12.2 Ascending input from the lung receptors

(a) is carried by the IX cranial nerve

(b) always depresses breathing

(c) is first received by the nucleus tractus solitarii

(d) is first received by the pneumotaxic centre

12.3 Stretch receptors in the lung

(a) are mostly rapidly adapting

(b) are responsible for the Hering–Breuer inspiratory reflex

(c) detect fluid accumulation in the lung interstitium

(d) are of limited importance in humans

12.4 Which of the following has NOT been implicated in the generation of basic respiratory rhythm?

(a) pre-Bötzinger complex

(b) a switching circuit between pons and medulla

(c) dorsal respiratory group

(d) the pyramidal tracts

Chapter 13: Pulmonary circulation and anatomical right-to-left shunts

13.1 Compared to the systemic circulation, the pulmonary circulation

(a) has less pulsatile flow in the capillaries

(b) has total resistance which is about one-third that of the systemic circulation

(c) lacks autoregulation of blood flow

(d) is strongly controlled by autonomic nerves

13.2 The forces affecting fluid movement across the pulmonary capillaries

(a) result in net absorption in normal pulmonary capillaries

(b) are reduced lying down

(c) favour increased filtration in a patient with severe mitral stenosis

(d) favour increased filtration in a patient with severe pulmonary stenosis

13.3 All of the following are examples of conditions that usually give a pure right-to-left shunt EXCEPT:

(a) atrial septal defect

(b) lobar pneumonia

(c) tetralogy of Fallot

(d) atelectasis

13.4 Some right-to-left shunting occurs in healthy people

(a) because there is usually some areas of unventilated alveoli

(b) because all of the venous blood from the bronchial circulation drains into the pulmonary veins

(c) because all of the venous blood from the ventricular myocardium drains into the pulmonary veins

(d) and is the main reason why arterial PO_2 is always less than pulmonary capillary PO_2

Chapter 14: Ventilation–perfusion mismatching

14.1 In a person with ventilation–perfusion mismatching

(a) regions with ventilation–perfusion ratios of 0.3 are dead-space effect regions

(b) regions with high ventilation–perfusion ratios have equal and opposite effects on arterial PCO_2 and PO_2 as regions with low ventilation–perfusion ratios

(c) regions with low ventilation–perfusion ratios are the main cause of cyanosis in a patient with a severe asthma attack

(d) the effects on arterial PO_2 and PCO_2 are usually quite different from those of a pure right-to-left shunt

14.2 Oxygen-enriched inspired air

(a) can significantly improve oxygen saturation of the blood emerging from regions with some ventilation but a low ventilation–perfusion ratio

(b) is more likely to reverse the cyanosis of a patient with tetralogy of Fallot than that of an asthmatic patient with severe ventilation–perfusion mismatching

(c) will cause pulmonary blood vessels to dilate

(d) can significantly improve oxygen saturation of blood emerging from regions with high ventilation–perfusion ratio

14.3 In a young asthmatic patient with arterial hypoxia during a severe attack

(a) the arterial PCO_2 would be expected to be high

(b) a low arterial PCO_2 would be expected but if high would not be an important problem

(c) a low arterial PCO_2 would be expected and if normal (5.3 kPa, 40 mmHg) or high would be cause for concern

(d) 24% oxygen is the appropriate inspired gas

14.4 The A–a PO_2 gradient

(a) is the difference between the PO_2 in the alveolar gas and in the blood at the end of the pulmonary capillary

(b) is normally about 5 kPa (37.5 mmHg) in a young person

(c) is increased by hypoventilation

(d) is usually increased by either right-to-left shunts or ventilation–perfusion mismatching

Chapter 15: Exercise, altitude and diving

15.1 In exercise, as the work load increases progressively

(a) the oxygen extraction increases progressively until at maximum exercise all the oxygen has been removed from the venous blood

(b) arterial PCO_2 is little changed in mild to moderate exercise but falls in heavy exercise

(c) alveolar ventilation approximately doubles when the carbon dioxide production has risen fourfold

(d) the main determinant of the maximum oxygen uptake that a person can achieve is his/her maximum ventilation

15.2 On acute ascent to high altitude

(a) ventilation rises to about four times the sea level value at 3000 m (10 000 ft)

(b) high altitude pulmonary oedema only occurs in patients with heart failure

(c) a rise in haemoglobin concentration occurs and improves tissue oxygenation

(d) hypoxic pulmonary vasoconstriction occurs but is of little benefit at altitude

15.3 A person travels from sea level to an altitude of 4000 m (13 000 ft). A week after arriving

(a) arterial P_{CO_2} is higher than on the day of arrival

(b) the rise in haemoglobin concentration has reached a plateau

(c) any symptoms of acute mountain sickness are likely to have improved

(d) arterial PO_2 will have returned to the sea level value

15.4 During diving

(a) descending rapidly while holding your breath may cause lung rupture

(b) nitrogen narcosis is a potential problem when breathing compressed air

(c) decompression sickness is due to bubbles of CO_2 forming in the tissues

(d) breathing air through a long tube open at the surface of the water is an alternative to using compressed gas during dives up to 5 m below the surfaces

Chapter 16: Development of the respiratory system and birth

16.1 Airway smooth muscle

(a) originates from the primitive endoderm of foregut

(b) originates from splanchnic mesoderm

(c) is mostly formed during the pseudoglandular period

(d) does not appear in terminal bronchioles until after birth

16.2 The lung increases in size over the first 3 years after birth

(a) as a result of branching morphogenesis

(b) until there are about 30 generations of airways

(c) largely due to increased number of alveoli and respiratory bronchioles

(d) due to growth of airway smooth muscle and cartilage

16.3 The P_aO_2 of fetal blood

(a) maintains the patency of the ductus arteriosus

(b) is independent of the maternal P_aO_2

(c) is maintained by a special (fetal) form of haemoglobin

(d) is about 8 kPa

16.4 At birth

(a) the rapid rise in P_aO_2 initiates closure of the ductus venosus

(b) the foramen ovale only closes some days after birth

(c) fluid in the lungs is expelled by rhythmic contraction of airway smooth muscle

(d) surfactant is essential for expansion of the alveoli

Chapter 17: Complications of development and congenital disease

17.1 Neonatal respiratory distress syndrome (NRDS)

(a) occurs in ~50% of premature births with a weight of <1500 g

(b) always following premature births before 30-week gestation

(c) is commonly treated by giving the neonate corticosteroids

(d) occurs in 1 in 300 of all births

17.2 Which of the following congenital diseases affecting the lung is most common?

(a) lack of pulmonary surfactant protein B

(b) tracheo-oesophageal fistula

(c) congenital diaphragmatic hernia

(d) Marfan's disease

17.3 Which option is NOT correct concerning oesophageal atresia?

(a) It leads to distension of the gut with air.

(b) It is commonly associated with polyhydramnios.

(c) It is associated with 85% of cases of tracheo-oesophageal fistula.

(d) It originates in the 10th week of development.

17.4 Bronchopulmonary dysplasia

(a) is primarily caused by medical treatment of premature neonates

(b) can be minimized by ventilation with high O_2 immediately after birth

(c) is invariably fatal within 2 years

(d) is due to a genetic defect of lung development

Chapter 18: Lung defence mechanisms and immunology

18.1 Physical defences in the upper airways

(a) include cilia in the nasopharynx that catch large particles

(b) prevent particles greater than 1 μm entering the bronchi

(c) include humidification of air to prevent the epithelium from drying out

(d) are independent of mucus

18.2 Mucus

(a) contains immunoglobulins of which IgM is the most prevalent

(b) consists largely of glycoproteins

(c) is secreted by squamous epithelial cells in the lower airways

(d) acts as a purely passive barrier and transport mechanism

18.3 Removal of invading materials/organisms from the alveoli

(a) requires mucociliary transport

(b) is dependent on phagocytosis by macrophages

(c) is enhanced by coughing

(d) requires infiltration of plasma cells

18.4 Which form of immunoglobulin is secreted across the epithelium?

(a) IgE

(b) IgG

(c) IgA

(d) IgM

Chapter 19: History and examination

19.1 What is the most common cause of haemoptysis?

(a) lung infarction

(b) bronchial carcinoma

(c) pulmonary vasculitis

(d) infections

19.2 On examination of the hands of a patient with type 2 respiratory failure, which of the following would be most common?

(a) finger clubbing

(b) fine tremor

(c) clammy skin

(d) coarse tremor

19.3 On auscultation of the patient's chest you hear fine inspiratory crackles; with which condition is this most often associated?

(a) asthma

(b) lung consolidation

(c) interstitial fibrosis

(d) emphysema

19.4 The sound on percussion of a patient's chest is hyperresonant; which condition might this reflect?

(a) asthma or COPD

(b) pneumothorax

(c) interstitial fibrosis

(d) emphysema

Chapter 20: Pulmonary function tests

20.1 When trying to determine whether a breathless patient has obstructive or restrictive pulmonary disease

    (a) it is necessary to make measurements of airway resistance and lung compliance

    (b) a peak expiratory flow rate above the predicted value indicates restrictive disease

    (c) the most useful test is the forced expiratory spirogram (exhaled volume vs time)

    (d) inspiratory wheezing would be expected in obstructive pulmonary disease

20.2 Forced expiratory volume in 1 second (FEV$_1$)

    (a) increases with age until a person stops growing when he/she is about 18 years old

    (b) remains at the same level once it has reached its peak value provided that the person does not smoke or develop a respiratory disease

    (c) if its value in litres is reduced but it is normal as a percentage of the subject's forced vital capacity ($>75\%$ FVC), it indicates restrictive lung disease

    (d) is not greatly affected by the subject's effort and technique

20.3 The best single measurement indicating a respiratory problem and which is reproducible and best correlates with function and prognosis is

    (a) forced expiratory volume in 1 second, FEV$_1$

    (b) forced vital capacity, FVC

    (c) peak expiratory flow rate, PEFR

    (d) maximal voluntary ventilation, MVV

20.4 In patients with restrictive ventilatory defects

    (a) a high transdiaphragmatic pressure would suggest respiratory muscle weakness

    (b) a normal K_{CO} ($= D_L CO/V_A$) suggests a cause outside the lungs such as respiratory muscle weakness

    (c) resting hypoxia can be expected when D_{LCO} is 50% predicted

    (d) functional residual capacity is very low in patients with respiratory muscle weakness

Chapter 21: Chest imaging and bronchoscopy

21.1 A routine screening chest X-ray (CXR)

    (a) always includes a lateral CXR

    (b) is performed at full expiration

    (c) allows visualization of the mediastinum

    (d) with anterior–posterior (AP) films allow a detailed view of lung parenchyma

21.2 Which of the following is NOT normally an indication for computed tomography?

    (a) pleural disease

    (b) pulmonary vasculitis

    (c) pulmonary emboli

    (d) parenchymal disease

21.3 What is the gold standard for diagnosing pulmonary emboli?

    (a) ventilation–perfusion scans

    (b) High-resolution computed tomography

    (c) positron emission tomography

    (d) pulmonary angiography

21.4 Bronchoscopy

    (a) is most commonly performed under general anaesthesia

    (b) allows visualization down to the third and fourth divisions of the endobronchial tree

    (c) can be used in the diagnosis of parenchymal lung disease

    (d) commonly causes cardiac arrhythmias

Chapter 22: Public health and smoking

22.1 Respiratory disease

    (a) accounts for 10% of all deaths in the UK

    (b) accounts for 5% of emergency hospital admissions

    (c) due to emphysema causes reduced exercise tolerance in 1 million people in the USA

    (d) accounts for $\sim$100 000 hospital admissions per year in the UK

22.2 Smoking-related disease

    (a) accounts for $\sim$20% of all deaths in the UK

    (b) is the second greatest cause of preventable illness and mortality worldwide

    (c) is largely restricted to respiratory problems

    (d) is decreasing worldwide

22.3 Progressive decline in lung function (FEV$_1$)

    (a) ceases on stopping smoking

    (b) does not occur in healthy non-smokers

    (c) causes disability when the FEV$_1$ falls to about 25% of that at 25 years old

    (d) is strongly accelerated in all smokers

22.4 Smoking cessation

    (a) reduces the risk of lung cancer to that in non-smokers

    (b) causes an increase in brain dopamine

    (c) rates are improved most by treatment with bupropion

    (d) rates are improved by decreasing the reward effects with partial agonists of nicotinic acetylcholine receptors

Chapter 23: Respiratory failure

23.1 Hypercapnia is in inevitable when the cause of hypoxia is

    (a) ventilation–perfusion mismatching

    (b) diffusion impairment

    (c) hypoventilation

    (d) low inspired PO_2

23.2 Respiratory failure

    (a) is present and known as 'type 1' in a patient with an arterial PO_2 of 7 kPa (53 mmHg) and a PCO_2 of 4 kPa (30 mmHg)

    (b) is present in a patient disabled by breathlessness at rest, with an arterial PO_2 of 9 kPa

    (c) is classed as type 2 if P_aCO_2 is high but PO_2 is normal

    (d) nearly always requires some kind of mechanical ventilatory support

23.3 Typical symptoms and signs caused by a high P_aCO_2 include

    (a) cold pale skin

    (b) weak pulse

    (c) headache, which is often worse following sleep

    (d) central cyanosis

23.4 Chronic arterial hypoxia combined with chronic arterial hypercapnia

    (a) is often associated with anaemia

    (b) could explain an arterial pH of 7.2 because of the high arterial PCO_2

(c) is a typical finding in patients with a right-to-left shunt due to cyanotic heart disease (e.g. tetralogy of Fallot)

(d) is commonly complicated by pulmonary hypertension

Chapter 24: Asthma: pathophysiology

24.1 Which of the following is NOT a characteristic of asthma?

(a) increase in IgG immunoglobulins

(b) airway hyperresponsiveness

(c) infiltration of eosinophils into the airways

(d) increased mucus production

24.2 The most common allergens associated with asthma in the UK are (in order of importance)

(a) pollens; house dust mite; fungal spores

(b) house dust mite; pollens; animal dander

(c) house dust mite; pollens; fungal spores

(d) house dust mite; animal dander; pollens

24.3 The immediate response of asthma involves

(a) mast cell degranulation

(b) binding of antigen to IgE on macrophages

(c) release of cytokines such as IL-13

(d) activation of cholinergic nerves

24.4 Chronic asthma is associated with:

(a) activation of eosinophils

(b) activation of T_{H1} lymphocytes

(c) reduced function of goblet cells

(d) decreased permeability of submucosal capillaries

Chapter 25: Asthma: treatment

25.1 Which test is NOT used during diagnosis or monitoring of asthma?

(a) diffusing capacity

(b) peak expiratory flow rate

(c) bronchial challenge test

(d) skin prick test

25.2 Which drug is the most commonly prescribed preventer therapy in asthma?

(a) β_2-adrenoreceptor agonists

(b) xanthines such as theophylline

(c) muscarinic receptor antagonists

(d) inhaled steroids

25.3 Long-acting β_2-adrenoreptor agonists

(a) work by increasing cGMP in airway smooth muscle

(b) may become less efficacious due to tolerance after long-term use

(c) can be used as the sole therapy in asthma

(d) are the first choice for a reliever therapy

25.4 Which of the following is NOT a common adverse effect of low-dose inhaled steroids?

(a) cough

(b) weight gain

(c) oral candidiasis

(d) hoarseness

Chapter 26: Chronic obstructive pulmonary disease

26.1 Which of the following is NOT normally associated with chronic bronchitis?

(a) increased total lung capacity

(b) Co_2 retention

(c) less than 15% increase in FEV_1 following treatment with a bronchodilator or steroids

(d) polycythaemia

26.2 Which of the following is NOT normally associated with emphysema?

(a) decreased D_LCO (diffusion capacity)

(b) increased residual volume

(c) cyanosis at rest

(d) hyperinflation

26.3 Why do patients with emphysema often exhibit purse-lipped breathing?

(a) chest discomfort during inspiration

(b) regulates filling of lungs that have increased compliance

(c) increases airway pressure during expiration to reduce air trapping

(d) reflex response to severe breathlessness

26.4 Which of the following statements about COPD is NOT true?

(a) It can be caused by α_1-antitrypsin deficiency.

(b) Bronchodilators such as β-agonists never improve symptoms or lung function.

(c) Patients may benefit from flu vaccinations.

(d) Surgical reduction of lung volume may be useful in advanced disease.

Chapter 27: Pulmonary hypertension

27.1 Pulmonary hypertension is defined as

(a) a mean pulmonary artery pressure (PAP) >25 mmHg during exercise

(b) a mean PAP ~15 mmHg at rest that increases to >20 mmHg during exercise

(c) a mean PAP >25 mmHg at rest or >30 mmHg during exercise

(d) a mean PAP > 90 mmHg at rest or > 110 mmHg during exercise

27.2 The most common cause of pulmonary hypertension is

(a) hypoxaemia secondary to respiratory diseases

(b) left heart failure

(c) pulmonary embolism

(d) genetic defects

27.3 Idiopathic pulmonary arterial hypertension

(a) commonly causes pulmonary oedema

(b) is most prevalent in women aged 40 years or more

(c) has a mean survival without treatment of 2 years

(d) occurs in 1 per 100 000 population

27.4 Which of the following drugs is NOT used for treatment of pulmonary hypertension?

(a) sildenafil (type 5 phosphodiesterase inhibitor)

(b) bosentan (endothelin receptor antagonist)

(c) prostacyclin analogues (increases cAMP)

(d) fenfluramine (modulates serotonin uptake and release)

Chapter 28: Venous thromboembolism and pulmonary embolism

28.1 Deep vein thrombosis

(a) propagating into the femoral and iliac veins has a 50% chance of causing pulmonary embolism

(b) occurs in 50% of patients undergoing hip or knee replacement surgery in the absence of prophylactic therapy

(c) is most likely to form an embolus once the thrombus is organized

(d) is commonly treated with thrombolytic agents

28.2 Pulmonary embolism

(a) causes an increase in lung dead space

(b) has a mortality of 25%

(c) commonly causes hypercapnia and hypoxaemia

(d) always reduces cardiac output

28.3 The diagnostic standard for pulmonary embolism is

(a) chest X-ray

(b) V/Q scanning

(c) pulmonary angiography

(d) spiral/helical computed tomography

28.4 Standard treatment for pulmonary embolism is

(a) immediate thrombolytics

(b) warfarin, continued for 3–6 months

(c) initially heparin, followed by warfarin for 3–6 months

(d) heparin until the embolism resolves

Chapter 29: Pulmonary vasculitis

29.1 Pulmonary vasculitis

(a) rarely involves other vascular beds

(b) is primarily associated with inflammation and necrosis of the blood vessels

(c) is the most common manifestation of rheumatoid arthritis in the lung

(d) is mostly caused by infection

29.2 Which of the following is NOT a primary vasculitides?

(a) Churg–Strauss syndrome

(b) Wegener's granulomatosis

(c) Goodpasture's syndrome

(d) systemic lupus erythematosus

29.3 Which of the following is NOT normally associated with vasculitides?

(a) Increased anti-neutrophil cytoplasmic antibodies (ANCA)

(b) capillary rupture and alveolar haemorrhage

(c) hypoxaemia

(d) infiltration of eosinophils

29.4 What is the most common therapy for pulmonary vasculitis?

(a) inhaled low-dose corticosteroids

(b) chemotherapy

(c) oral corticosteroids

(d) plasmapheresis

Chapters 30 and 31: Diffuse parenchymal (interstitial) lung diseases/Sarcoidosis

30.1 The most common form of DPLD is

(a) occupational lung disease

(b) sarcoidosis

(c) idiopathic interstitial pneumonitis

(d) drug induced

30.2 DPLD is commonly associated with

(a) increased lung compliance

(b) an obstructive defect

(c) decreased $D_L CO$

(d) increased residual volume

30.3 The most frequent form of non-usual interstitial pneumonitis is

(a) non-specific interstitial pneumonitis (NSIP)

(b) cryptogenic organizing pneumonia (COP)

(c) hypersensitivity pneumonitis

(d) lymphoid interstitial pneumonitis (LIP)

30.4 Which of the following is least likely to respond to treatment with steroids?

(a) non-specific interstitial pneumonitis (NSIP)

(b) desquamative interstitial pneumonitis (DIP)

(c) sarcoidosis

(d) usual interstitial pneumonia (UIP)

Chapter 32: Pleural diseases

32.1 Pleurisy

(a) is a common term used for all diseases of the pleura

(b) is due to inflammation of the pleura

(c) is made worse by deep inspiration

(d) is not present in pneumothorax

32.2 The fluid between the parietal and visceral pleurae

(a) is normally protein-rich

(b) is primarily drained by the visceral lymphatics

(c) is formed by net filtration of a transudative fluid

(d) has a volume of >300 mL

32.3 Exudative pleural effusions

(a) are protein-poor

(b) are always associated with infection

(c) are mostly commonly caused by congestive heart failure

(d) often have raised lactate dehydrogenase

32.4 Mesothelioma

(a) has a median survival of >5 years

(b) most commonly occurs 5–10 years after asbestos exposure

(c) is invariably fatal

(d) can be treated with steroids

Chapter 33: Occupational and environmental-related lung disease

33.1 The most common form of occupational and environmental lung disease

(a) is due to atmospheric pollution and secondary smoking

(b) causes lung fibrosis

(c) is triggered as a result of workplace substances in 10 000 people in the UK per year

(d) is asthma

33.2 Which of the following statements about inhaled irritants is UNTRUE?

(a) Highly soluble agents (e.g. ammonia) favour damage to the alveolar epithelium.

(b) Extensive exposure can lead to bronchiolitis obliterans after 2–8 weeks.

(c) Activation of irritant receptors leads to dyspnoea.

(d) Diesel particulates increase mortality particularly in the elderly.

33.3 Pneumoconiosis

(a) is caused by inhalation of organic materials

(b) can in some cases develop into progressive massive fibrosis

(c) tends to result in reversible airways obstruction

(d) does not include asbestosis

33.4 Which of the following statements about Farmer's lung is UNTRUE?

(a) It is the most common example of extrinsic allergic alveolitis.

(b) It is due to contamination with thermophilic actinomycetes bacteria.

(c) It can lead to interstitial fibrosis.

(d) Removal of exposure always results in rapid recovery.

Chapter 34: Cystic fibrosis and bronchiectasis

34.1 Cystic fibrosis is

(a) an autosomal dominant trait

(b) due to the ΔF508 mutation in <60% of cases

(c) associated with infertility in males more commonly than in females

(d) characterized by increased mucus production

34.2 The cystic fibrosis transmembrane conductance regulator (CFTR)

(a) is activated by cyclic guanine monophosphate

(b) is an epithelial sodium channel

(c) controls mucus hydration and viscosity

(d) is only present in the epithelium of the lower airways

34.3 The most important treatment for cystic fibrosis is

(a) to improve nutrition

(b) to control infection

(c) to promote mucus clearance

(d) to reduce inflammation

34.4 Which statement is NOT true concerning bronchiectasis?

(a) It is caused by persistent infection and inflammation in proximal bronchi.

(b) Finger clubbing is often seen in patients with bronchiectasis.

(c) Most cases in the UK are associated with cystic fibrosis.

(d) It can rarely be detected by radiographic imaging.

Chapter 35: Pneumothorax

35.1 A pneumothorax that causes mediastinal shift and compression of the functioning lung is called

(a) primary pneumothorax

(b) secondary pneumothorax

(c) traumatic pneumothorax

(d) tension pneumothorax

35.2 Primary pneumothorax

(a) occurs in 8 per 10^5 young men over 1.9 m in height in a year

(b) is the most common form of pneumothorax

(c) usually occurs when there is an underlying lung disease

(d) is caused by air leaking across the parietal pleura

35.3 A pneumothorax of <30%

(a) will always be aspirated whatever the type

(b) is generally asymptomatic

(c) usually requires hospital admission if it is secondary to respiratory disease

(d) is treated with pleurodesis

35.4 Secondary pneumothorax is a particular risk for

(a) mechanical ventilation for lung disease

(b) tuberculosis

(c) pneumonia

(d) asthma

Chapters 36 and 37: Community-acquired pneumonia/Hospital-acquired (nosocomial) pneumonia

36.1 Concerning community acquired pneumonia

(a) the incidence is 5–11 cases per 10 000 population

(b) the most frequently identified organisms are Gram-negative bacteria

(c) risk factors include age (<5, >65 years)

(d) symptoms always include pleurisy and haemoptysis

36.2 Concerning hospital acquired pneumonia

(a) incidence is 0.5–2% of all hospital patients

(b) the most frequently identified organism is *Streptococcus pneumonia*

(c) risk is doubled by mechanical ventilation

(d) treatment is the same as for community acquired pneumonia

36.3 Which of the following statements in NOT true concerning the management of pneumonia?

(a) CXR is used to confirm diagnosis.

(b) Antibiotics therapy should only start once the infecting organism is identified.

(c) Typical and atypical pneumonias are difficult to differentiate.

(d) O_2 therapy is commonly used to maintain S_aO_2 >90%.

36.4 Which of the following does NOT suggest increased risk of mortality in patients admitted to hospital for pneumonia?

(a) respiratory rate >30/min

(b) age >65 years

(c) mean blood pressure >110 mmHg

(d) urea >7 mmol/L

Chapter 38: Pulmonary tuberculosis

38.1 Which statement is INCORRECT concerning TB?

(a) Infection with TB is via inhalation.

(b) Susceptibility to TB is greater in the elderly.

(c) Infection results in formation of a granuloma.

(d) The Ghon focus is known as the primary complex.

38.2 Investigations of TB

(a) the Mantoux test is often negative in Miliary TB

(b) the Heaf test is the most commonly used test

(c) Miliary TB is easily detected by upper lobe shadowing in CXR

(d) *Mycobacterium tuberculosis* bacilli are acid-fast and grow rapidly

38.3 Which of the following is NOT a common feature of TB?

(a) erythema nodosum

(b) pleural effusions

(c) pulmonary oedema

(d) bronchiectasis

38.4 Treatment of TB

(a) corticosteroids are prescribed to all patients

(b) an important factor is patient compliance with therapy

(c) drug treatment is maintained for 2 months in uncomplicated cases

(d) Pyridoxine is given with isoniazid to limit liver dysfunction

Chapter 39: The immunocompromised host

39.1 Which of the following is NOT normally associated with immunosuppression?

(a) diabetes

(b) treatment with steroids

(c) smoking

(d) malnutrition

39.2 Which of the following is NOT a consequence of chemotherapy?

(a) neutropaenia

(b) impaired T-cell function

(c) complement deficiency

(d) increased susceptibility to fungal infections

39.3 The HIV-positive patient

(a) HIV causes depletion of CD4 T-lymphocytes

(b) the commonest chest infection is PCP (*Pneumocystis jirovecii pneumonia*)

(c) in the UK, 10% of cases with mycobacterium tuberculosis are co-infected with HIV

(d) *Cytomegalovirus* (CMV) infection is rare in HIV

39.4 Which statement is NOT true concerning identification of respiratory infections in the Immunocompromised host?

(a) Chest computed tomography can be diagnostic for aspergillosis.

(b) Early bronchoalveolar lavage can aid diagnosis in ~55% of cases.

(c) Pleural fluid is rarely investigated in such patients.

(d) CXR may show diffuse infiltrates but be otherwise non-specific.

Chapter 40: Lung cancer

40.1 Lung cancer

(a) has an overall 5-year survival of <15%

(b) has an increased risk of 5% due to passive smoking

(c) is likely to decrease in women over the next 10 years

(d) is most commonly caused in rural areas by natural radon gas

40.2 The least common type of lung cancer is:

(a) small cell

(b) squamous cell

(c) large cell

(d) adenocarcinoma

40.3 In the context of lung cancer, which of the following is NOT a paraneoplastic syndrome?

(a) Lambert–Eaton syndrome

(b) idiopathic orthostatic hypotension

(c) extrathoracic metastasis

(d) Cushing's syndrome

40.4 Staging for small cell cancer

(a) as *limited disease* predicts median survival of 5 years.

(b) as *extensive disease* describes metastatic spread beyond the hemithorax

(c) is similar to that for non-small cell cancer

(d) depends on the tumour, node and metastasis classification

Chapter 41: Acute respiratory distress syndrome

41.1 Which of the following is NOT part of the criteria for diagnosis of ARDS?

(a) severe hypoxaemia

(b) hypercapnia

(c) bilateral diffuse pulmonary infiltrates on chest X-ray

(d) near normal left atrial pressure

41.2 Which of the following statements about ARDS is true?

(a) The incidence of ARDS is only slightly less than that of acute lung injury.

(b) ARDS precipitated by sepsis has the greatest mortality.

(c) Most patients die from hypoxaemia alone.

(d) The primary defect is increased permeability of the alveolar–capillary membrane.

41.3 Clinical features of ARDS

(a) the acute inflammatory phase lasts 24 hours

(b) the late fibroproliferative phase is associated with multiorgan failure

(c) pneumothorax is common in the late fibroproliferative phase

(d) the combination of cyanosis, dyspnoea, confusion and lung crepitations is diagnostic

41.4 Which of the following is NOT generally beneficial in early ARDS?

(a) avoidance of excessive fluid loading

(b) treatment with steroids and other anti-inflammatory agents

(c) physiotherapy

(d) Non-invasive or full mechanical ventilation

Chapter 42: Mechanical ventilation

42.1 Mechanical ventilation

(a) is used more often for type 1 than type 2 respiratory failure

(b) will always be needed for a patient with a cervical cord transection at C7

(c) in non-surgical patients is increasingly being carried out using non-invasive techniques

(d) is relatively free from complications

42.2 In a paralysed patient on intermittent positive pressure ventilation (IPPV)

(a) inspiration is brought about by a fall in intrapleural and alveolar pressure

(b) if hypoxia occurs the tidal volume and respiratory frequency of the ventilator should be increased

(c) the usual settings include an inspiratory time which is longer than the expiratory time

(d) minute ventilation is usually adjusted to maintain a $P_a\text{CO}_2$ at a near normal level (~5 kPa, 37 mmHg)

42.3 Which statement is INCORRECT concerning continuous positive airway pressure (CPAP)?

(a) It can be used to take over the work of breathing.

(b) It is applied using a nasal or face mask.

(c) It can be used to prevent upper airways collapse in sleep apnoea.

(d) It can be used in interstitial diseases to reduce V_A/Q mismatch.

42.4 Non-invasive intermittent positive pressure ventilation, NIPPV,

(a) produces a similar airway pressure profile to the produced by a tank ventilator ('iron lung')

(b) helps reduce the work of breathing and is very useful for exhausted patients with respiratory failure

(c) is not a suitable technique for exacerbations of severe chronic obstructive pulmonary disease (COPD)

(d) is usually applied through an endotracheal tube

Chapter 43: Oxygenation and oxygen therapy

43.1 Tissue hypoxia

(a) occurs within 2 minutes of failure of ventilation

(b) is unlikely in patients with polycythaemia

(c) can be caused by CO poisoning

(d) only occurs when $S_a\text{O}_2$ is low

43.2 In O_2 therapy the initial target $S_a\text{O}_2$

(a) should always be less than 92% to prevent hypercapnia

(b) should be 88–92% in patients at risk of type 1 respiratory failure

(c) should always be as high as possible

(d) should be 88–92% in patients with high P_{CO_2} and bicarbonate but normal pH

43.3 Preferred method for O_2 delivery in patients at the risk of type 2 respiratory failure

(a) fixed performance Venturi mask with 24–28% O_2

(b) nasal cannulae with 40–60% O_2

(c) nasal cannulae with 24–28% O_2

(d) non-rebreathing reservoir mask with 24–28% O_2

43.4 Which is NOT a recognized risk for high-dose O_2 therapy?

(a) collapse of poorly ventilated airways

(b) adult respiratory distress syndrome (ARDS)

(c) pulmonary hypertension due to pulmonary artery constriction

(d) cerebral vasospasm or vasoconstriction

Chapter 44: Sleep apnoea

44.1 Which of the following is NOT commonly associated with sleep apnoea?

(a) daytime hypersomnolence

(b) increased risk of hypertension

(c) increased haemoglobin

(d) nocturia

44.2 Which statement is NOT true concerning obstructive sleep apnoea (OSA)?

(a) 90% of patients with sleep apnoea have OSA.

(b) OSA is associated with increased neck circumference.

(c) OSA is equally common in men and women.

(d) OSA is associated with REM sleep.

44.3 Which is generally the most long-term therapy for OSA?

(a) moderate weight loss

(b) nocturnal O_2 therapy

(c) nasal continuous positive airway pressure (CPAP)

(d) surgery

44.4 Central sleep apnoea

(a) is always due to a defect in the respiratory central pattern generator

(b) is always associated with daytime hypercapnia

(c) can occur during REM sleep in some patients with COPD

(d) can be effectively treated with CPAP

Answers

1.1: b;	1.2: c;	1.3: d;	1.4: a;
2.1: c;	2.2: a;	2.3: d;	2.4: a;
3.1: c;	3.2: b;	3.3: b;	3.4: c;
4.1: b;	4.2: d;	4.3: b;	4.4: c;
5.1: d;	5.2: c;	5.3: b;	5.4: b;
6.1: d;	6.2: d;	6.3: a;	6.4: c;
7.1: d;	7.2: b;	7.3: b;	7.4: c;
8.1: b;	8.2: d;	8.3: d;	8.4: a;
9.1: c;	9.2: d;	9.3: c;	9.4: d;
10.1: d;	10.2: a;	10.3: d;	10.4: c;
11.1: c;	11.2: c;	11.3: a;	11.4: c;
12.1: b;	12.2: c;	12.3: b;	12.4: d;
13.1: c;	13.2: c;	13.3: a;	13.4: d;
14.1: c;	14.2: a;	14.3: c;	14.4: a;
15.1: b;	15.2: d;	15.3: c;	15.4: b;
16.1: b;	16.2: c;	16.3: a;	16.4: d;
17.1: a;	17.2: c;	17.3: d;	17.4: a;
18.1: c;	18.2: b;	18.3: b;	18.4: c;
19.1: d;	19.2: d;	19.3: c;	19.4: b;
20.1: c;	20.2: c;	20.3: a;	20.4: b;
21.1: c;	21.2: b;	21.3: d;	21.4: c;
22.1: c;	22.2: a;	22.3: c;	22.4: d;
23.1: c;	23.2: a;	23.3: c;	23.4: d;
24.1: a;	24.2: b;	24.3: a;	24.4: a;
25.1: a;	25.2: d;	25.3: b;	25.4: b;
26.1: a;	26.2: c;	26.3: c;	26.4: b;
27.1: c;	27.2: a;	27.3: c;	27.4: d;
28.1: a;	28.2: a;	28.3: c;	28.4: c;
29.1: b;	29.2: d;	29.3: d;	29.4: c;
30.1: c;	30.2: c;	30.3: a;	30.4: d;
32.1: c;	32.2: c;	32.3: d;	32.4: c;
33.1: d;	33.2: a;	33.3: b;	33.4: d;
34.1: c;	34.2: c;	34.3: b;	34.4: d;
35.1: d;	35.2: b;	35.3: c;	35.4: a;
36.1: c;	36.2: a;	36.3: b;	36.4: c;
38.1: d;	38.2: a;	38.3: c;	38.4: b;
39.1: c;	39.2: c;	39.3: a;	39.4: c;
40.1: a;	40.2: c;	40.3: c;	40.4: b;
41.1: b;	41.2: d;	41.3: c;	41.4: b;
42.1: c;	42.2: d;	42.3: a;	42.4: b;
43.1: c;	43.2: d;	43.3: a;	43.4: c;
44.1: c;	44.2: c;	44.3: a;	44.4: c;

Index

Keep up with critical fields

Would you like to receive up-to-date information on our books, journals and databases in the areas that interest you, direct to your mailbox?

Join the **Wiley e-mail service** - a convenient way to receive updates and exclusive discount offers on products from us.

Simply visit www.wiley.com/email and register online

We won't bombard you with emails and we'll only email you with information that's relevant to you. We will ALWAYS respect your e-mail privacy and NEVER sell, rent, or exchange your e-mail address to any outside company. Full details on our privacy policy can be found online.

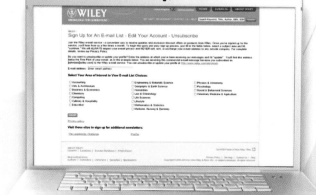

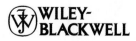
WILEY-BLACKWELL

www.wiley.com/email